Bill

Best wishes

Duane

THE
HEALTH CARE
SOLUTION

To the courageous people who are striving to find the best solutions to ensure that every American has equitable access to affordable, medically necessary quality health care.

THE HEALTH CARE SOLUTION

UNDERSTANDING THE CRISIS AND THE CURE

C. Duane Dauner
with
Michael Bowker

Vision Publishing
Sacramento, California

Published by: Vision Publishing
1201 K Street, Suite 800
Sacramento, CA 95814

Vision Publishing books may be purchased for educational, business, or sales promotional use. For information please write:
Special Marketing Department
Vision Publishing
1201 K Street, Suite 800
P.O. Box 1100
Sacramento, CA 95812-1100

Designed by Gary Hespenheide

Library of Congress Cataloging-in-Publication Data
Dauner, C. Duane
    The health care solution: understanding the crisis and the cure /
    C. Duane Dauner with Michael Bowker.—1st ed.
    p. cm.
    Pre-assigned LCCN: 93-060944
    ISBN 0-9636281-9-4
    1. Medical care—United States. 2. Medical care—United
    States—History. 3. Medical economics—United States.
    I. Bowker, Michael. II. Title
RA395.A3D38 1994
362.1'0973—QBI93-21568
10 9 8 7 6 5 4 3 2 1

First Edition

Printed in the United States of America

CONTENTS

ACKNOWLEDGMENTS

I am grateful to many people for their counsel, advice, and leadership during the past 27 years, and particularly during the last months of writing this book. They have helped me formulate the proposal that is offered in *The Health Care Solution.* The actual writing of the book is the culmination of this reflection and of my desire to help contribute to a better life for future generations. Any financial success from the book will benefit the Hospital Educational Foundation of California, a not-for-profit organization created by California hospitals to improve health care, provide education for the public and health professionals, assist in special research activities, and promote the general welfare.

I am indebted to several individuals for their assistance. Michael Bowker penned my ideas, thoughts and words in a coherent way. Gail Catlin guided the overall vision for the project. Lori Aldrete handled the management and coordination. Linda Allen pulled together the arrangements with the myriad details that are necessary in the production of a book. Michael Dimmitt reviewed the manuscript and coordinated much of the data that is included. David Iriguchi designed the graphs and charts.

It is my fortune to be involved in health care. Almost everyone I have encountered during my career has been sincere, honest, hardworking, and unselfish in their dedication to serve others. They have molded my thinking, and they are the lifeblood of *The Health Care Solution.*

C. Duane Dauner

FOREWORD

My father taught me as a young lad that "All politics is local," and saying that has been identified with me all my personal life.

It occurred to me that the saying could be tailored to describe this book: "All medical care is local." For Duane Dauner offers a health care plan that keeps its focus on the people. He is faithful to the precept that health care's overall mission is to serve individuals and society, as he says. In other words, "keep it on the local level."

If there is one fault I find with the medical profession it is that it has become too impersonal. It has gone from a profession in which success was measured by the quality of a doctor's bedside manner to one where success is determined by the bottom line. How cost effective is the treatment and how much will the traffic bear? What happened to compassion?

Duane adds: "Society, nevertheless, has a responsibility to provide for those who cannot provide for themselves." My philosophy exactly. I was pleased to see Duane state this principle, then propose a plan to ensure the least fortunate are covered.

During my 50 years in public service, I have seen few issues provoke the outcry that health care has in the last few years. Today, all Americans are troubled by our health care crisis. This is especially significant when we consider that there's no scarcity of issues to concern us. It is not often that our diverse society reaches consensus on complicated issues, but, as we saw during the 1992 presidential election, Americans of all social, economic, and political backgrounds want leadership in changing the health care system.

Since the mid-seventies, experts have known that, unless steps were taken to prevent it, a health care crisis in America was inevitable. Although the warnings were sounded, we as a nation failed to do anything substantial to avert the coming crisis. Certainly, some cautionary measures were taken. But, now it is evident that the "Band-aid" approach no longer suffices. We do not have the luxury of inaction for another twenty years. The problem is developing and implementing a plan for health care reform. President Clinton has proposed The Health Security Act and others have come forward with competing plans. Now that significant changes are on the horizon, both policy makers and the public will need the guidance and insight of thoughtful observers familiar with our health care system. This book will become one of those invaluable resources.

As president and CEO of the California Association of Hospitals and Health Systems, Duane has experienced firsthand this country's health care triumphs and shortcomings. Because he has spent more than 25 years in health care, he understands the system's ailments and explains why we must alter the way health care is perceived, delivered, and funded in this country.

I am delighted that Duane is sharing his vision for reform with those who most seek and deserve real answers—the American people. As you read on, I think you will agree that Duane's bold vision must be addressed if the necessary fundamental changes are to occur.

As a Congressman, I was always sensitive to the public's demand for specific solutions on issues that affect us all so deeply. Unfortunately, the specifics of health care are not easily determined.

Although there is no shortage of complaints about our health care problem, there is a scarcity of workable solutions to it. It is the objectivity in the book that makes *The Health Care Solution* so important.

Americans who want to know the whole story, so they can make informed decisions, will find it here. Beginning with a detailed look at the history of health care in America, Duane provides step-by-step guidelines for making needed changes. It is a plan that promises to be beneficial for patients, doctors, insurers and the government. Although we can learn from other countries' systems, America is so different that it is unrealistic to think that another system can merely be installed here. The plan outlined in these pages has been carefully crafted for our country's needs.

Like most Americans, I, too, am concerned about the quality, accessibility, and cost of health care on a personal level. I want to ensure that my family members receive the care they need in the years to come. With that in mind, I know we need to proceed rapidly—but cautiously—with real reform. This book contributes greatly toward that end.

Tip O'Neill
Speaker
U.S. House of Representatives (Retired)

INTRODUCTION

▼

Growing up in rural Kansas, my knowledge of health care was defined by what I experienced at the area 20-bed and 8-bed hospitals. The latter was run by a kindly physician and his R.N. wife who was the director of nursing. I remember them for their compassion and expert care. It would be some time before the importance of their efforts sank in, but when it did, it became evident that they had unwittingly formed my understanding of what caring and good health care are and should always be.

In 1965, I was a faculty member at Washburn University in Topeka embarking on an expected lifelong journey down the path of academia. At one of the usual faculty gatherings, I encountered a gentleman who chaired the Kansas Hospital Association and served on the American Hospital Association Board of Trustees, in addition to being on the university's board of regents. He pointed out the significance of health care and encouraged me to consider a career in the field, noting the unique challenges and rewards. My interest was piqued, and so I put my academic career on hold. After a little investigation, an important realization hit me: Few components of society are as valuable as health care.

In 1966, a scenario I witnessed at a hospital in western Kansas confirmed my finding. I was at the hospital to deliver a presentation and, after doing so, was given one of the hospital beds to sleep in for the night. About midnight, an ambulance brought in the victim of a severe auto accident. His condition was acute and his family was distraught. The hospital staff went to work trying to save him and simultaneously comfort his family. The speed with which they adroitly performed complicated procedures and the way they cared for his relatives—who, of course, were complete strangers—made a lasting impression on me. The next morning, I left the hospital knowing why health care transcends so many other services.

Some months later, I had to decide whether to remain in the health field or return to my academic pursuits. Around the same time, I met with Dr. Karl Menninger, who, incidently, is credited with developing the field of modern psychiatry. Upon hearing what was on my mind, he reminded me that truly great accomplishments generally are not fully achieved by individuals in their lifetimes. Encouraged by his comment, I realized that health care is not a lifelong job—it's a lifetime experience. After reflecting on my brief work in health care, it became obvious that I could make a more significant contribution to society by staying in the health field than by returning to academia.

Now, timing, the opportunities for reforms, and the beliefs that I have developed over all the years compelled me to write this book. My goal is to explain how health care in America became what it is today and where it is headed. You will find that detailed explanation in the following pages, as well as what I believe is a practical, fair plan for reform. As you begin to read, you may notice that this plan assigns the federal government a policy and supportive role. There are a few good reasons for this, the first of which is significant.

Several of the government's well-intentioned acts have contributed to our current health care troubles. Perhaps the most significant was the passage of Medicare and Medicaid in 1965. The legislation entitled the poor and elderly to "mainstream" health care—an undeniably humane and honorable goal. However, these laws successful by many measures, have contributed to the system's problems. This is primarily because the government failed to accurately estimate the way demographics and health care needs, technology and expectations might change in the future. As a result, when the increase in the average American's lifespan occurred (due in part to welcome medical advances) and we discovered that the growing elderly population consumed more services than any other group, it was a staggering blow because the government's financial projections fell way short of the actual expenditures. Now, the public views Medicare and Medicaid as a right, despite the government's unwillingness to pay the bill.

The government's management of medical education and the research boom also had an undesirable effect. One result of the vast increase in medical research was the influx of specialists it spawned. Because of this excess of specialists, we now have a shortage of generalist doctors. This is particularly alarming when we consider that generalist physicians are capable of meeting up to 75 percent of the public's needs.

Although the government has played a major part in creating the system's problems, we as providers, individuals, and a society also are at fault. Around the middle of the century, our attitude about health care began to shift. As a nation, we began to believe that everyone should have everything whenever it might be of some benefit. In conjunction with the medical advance boom, we imposed no limits on our self-defined "needs." Providers began to offer every imaginable service to remain competitive. Now, as a consequence, health care has fallen from its proper place in society. We all know that it can be one of the most constructive aspects of society, but because of the setbacks that have taken place in the last few decades, this, sadly, is no longer true. In order to return to the right perspective, we need to look at the elements that foster unnecessary use and make a concerted effort to optimize health care in an economic manner.

With so many forces coming to a head, now is the time to enact substantial change—before the opportunity passes. The plan proposed in this book incorporates many changes, but the first steps are restructuring the incentives that drive the system and realigning the way we view health care. Clearly, when we consider all the complex elements that will take great effort to fix, we also must change those that we control—such as our unhealthful habits and misuse of services.

Health reform is already occurring on a daily basis in an evolutionary way, as is indicated by the success of competitive alternatives such as integrated systems, health delivery networks and health maintenance organizations. However, the reforms are limited and unbalanced because they are not guided by a comprehensive plan and agreed upon goals. Naturally occurring reform is relevant because it signifies that change is inevitable, whether or not we participate in its creation or implementation.

Taking all this into consideration, I cannot over-emphasize the importance that the plan for reform be based in the people, not the federal government. We must be responsible for guiding the fundamental, philosophical, and structural changes. And if we act now, some of the values that are most important to us are more likely to survive the campaign for improvement. If we concede to apathy or frustration, we are sure to look back on this time with deep regret. *The Health Care Solution* is designed to give concerned citizens the information they need to act as reform gets underway. Of course, the government's support will be essential to the successful implementation of any universal reform measure. But its participation should be limited to providing authority and policy support; government must not be allowed to create, implement and control the plan.

Limiting the government's role in reform is critical to long-term success. Governmental control—especially in matters as seminal to our well-being as health care—is counter to our national consciousness and probably will be met with resistance in the one-to-one interactions of health care. In addition, government has a long history of enacting policy that contradicts the goals and values it espouses. Consider, for example, that although the U.S. surgeon general's office issues warnings on the known ills from tobacco, the federal government subsidizes those who grow it. That's like telling citizens not to drive more than 55 miles per hour, but subsidizing the fastest vehicles that can be produced. Regardless of the reasons for such contradictory behavior, the reality is that government is ill-equipped to remedy the system's complex problems and, therefore, should not micromanage reform.

The plan presented here is a compilation of previously introduced ideas and proposals, blended with new concepts to ensure successful implementation. The plan builds on Dr. Alain Enthoven's concept of managed competition, which was initially introduced in the late eighties, and on the health maintenance organizations' practice of using incentives and negotiated capitation payments for a designated set of services. Added to this are two more elements: 1) the bundling of payments so that insurance carriers and providers are integrated and consolidated, instead of being juxtaposed against each other, and 2) identifying inconsistencies between governmental policies and rhetoric. It is balanced to appeal to all stakeholders in a practical way.

My intent is that citizens understand the problems and possibilities associated with reforming our system. Such details are not readily understandable and people need the right information to make informed choices. It is my hope that you will take the information you are about to read and incorporate it into your discussions on health reform with friends and family. When given the chance, I hope you will also share your thoughts on this material with political representatives and health care professionals—whether it is on the local, state, or federal level.

Whatever your views, the time you spend on health reform could not be better spent. The price of inaction will far exceed the cost of constructively reforming the health care system now.

UNDERSTANDING THE CHANGE

The public is ready to make the hard choices in health care that their elected leaders are not.

—POLLSTER GEORGE GALLUP

To middle-income Americans, health care is a leading cause of personal bankruptcy and a source of constant anxiety. To the poor, health care is a fading dream. To the leaders of the most powerful country on earth, it is an unholy grail—a socioeconomic nightmare that gobbled up over $800 billion in 1992, even though more than 36 million Americans had no health coverage. However,

10 million of the uninsured had incomes of more than $30,000 per year. Nearly as many residents have inadequate health insurance.

National health expenditures
United States: Select Years 1960-1992* (000,000,000)

Year	Total Health Expenditure
1960	$ 27.1
1965	41.6
1970	74.4
1975	132.9
1980	250.1
1985	422.6
1990	675.0
1991	751.8
1992	819.9*

* Projected

SOURCE: Suzanne W. Letsch, et al., *Health Care Financing Review*, "National Health Expenditures, 1991," winter, 1992, Health Care Financing Administration, Baltimore, 1993. Sally T. Burner, et al., *Health Care Financing Review*, "National Health Expenditures through 2030," fall, 1992, Health Care Financing Administration, Baltimore, 1993.

Nonelderly population without health insurance by family income
United States: 1992

Family Income	Population Without Health Insurance 1992
Less than $5,000	4,400,000
$ 5,000-$ 9,999	5,100,000
$10,000-$14,999	5,600,000
$15,000-$19,999	4,700,000
$20,000-$29,999	6,600,000
$30,000-$39,999	3,800,000
$40,000-$49,999	2,400,000
$50,000 and Over	3,800,000
TOTAL	**36,300,000**

SOURCE: Employee Benefit Research Institute, *Special Report*, "Sources of Health Insurance and Characteristics of the Uninsured," Issue Brief Number 193, January 1993, Washington D.C.

From a service and technological standpoint, the United States health care industry remains the finest in the world. New medical breakthroughs are reported almost daily as the application of high-tech advancements such as lasers, computers, and telecommunications are blended with quantum leaps in medical intelligence. Yet, this entire glittering superstructure of accomplishment depends on a hopelessly antiquated and dangerously inadequate funding and delivery system. In a sense, what we have is a new Ferrari with bald tires and no brakes. We must either invest the time and resources necessary to fix the system, or face serious consequences.

In 1992, the U.S. spent nearly 14 percent of its gross domestic product (GDP) on health care. At the current rate of increase, that figure could leap above 18 percent by the end of the decade. It is unlikely the nation can sustain such a burden without severe economic and social repercussions. It is already damaging U.S. companies' ability to compete globally. General Motors, the largest employer-payer of health care in the nation, pays nearly $5 per hour per employee for health care, according to Richard O'Brien, vice president of corporate personnel. "We have to charge an additional $1,400 per vehicle to cover health care costs," says O'Brien. In Japan, the mark-up to cover health care costs amounts to less than $500 per vehicle.

The problem has hardly gone unrecognized. It was one of the critical issues in the 1992 presidential campaign and has triggered an avalanche of potential solutions. Unfortunately, many have proved more confusing than illuminating. Some are of questionable long-term value, others could prove to be counterproductive. A few move toward meeting the basic goals of universal access, a uniform benefit package, quality, economic discipline and

predictability, tax code revisions, and incentives, but none
put all of the essential components into a consistent, coherent plan.

Health as a percent of GDP
United States: Select Years 1960-1991 – Projections 1992-2030

Year	Percent
1960	5.3%
1965	5.9
1970	7.4
1975	8.4
1980	9.2
1985	10.5
1986	10.7
1987	10.9
1988	11.1
1989	11.5
1990	12.2
1991	13.2
1992*	13.9
1993*	14.4
1995*	15.6
2000*	18.1
2010*	22.0
2020*	26.5
2030*	32.0

* Projected data

SOURCE: United States Department of Health and Human Services, Health Care Financing
Administration, Office of the Actuary: Data from the Office of National Health Statistics.

Moreover, they fail to strike at the heart of the problem—the governmental command-and-control approach
to funding and delivery, which has caused the wasteful
horizontal expansion and overuse and duplication of
resources and technology. Any successful repair of the system must begin by replacing the conflicting and counterproductive incentives, which cause greater utilization of
services, more buildings and equipment, and a constant
pressure to work around regulations and controls.

MAKING THE HARD CHOICES

This book is not about a cosmetic reorganization of the health care system. It is, instead, a blueprint for fundamentally changing the way health care has historically been funded and delivered.

This book is about making difficult choices. It won't please everybody, especially those benefiting from the system's inefficiencies. The plan calls on interactive market forces, not government intervention, to control costs; it requires a complete restructuring. It requires government to change the way it thinks about health providers and alters the roles of the providers themselves. It requires health care users—all of us—to become more responsible in our demands and in the way we use the system. Most important, it calls for a harmonious alignment of the goals and incentives of government, health providers, payers, and users.

Finally, the book provides a plan of action for making these changes a reality, with an eye on the ultimate purpose—providing high-quality affordable health care to each American.

To understand the change, and the hard choices that lie ahead, it is imperative that we understand the volatile policy decisions and economic forces that ignited in the 1980s and 1990s and sent the American health care system careening off course.

A little history is in order.

A PROBLEM OF COST

America's health care system has two primary problems— access and cost. Simply put, open-ended health services cost more than the country is willing to pay. The result is a lack of access for millions of people and limited access for millions more.

Some of the reasons for the escalating cost, like America's aging population, cannot be mitigated, although they must be recognized. Our ever-increasing ability to prevent, diagnose, treat and cure diseases has greatly extended life expectancy in the U.S., but it has also created chaos for medicine and governmental programs.

In 1935, when Congress passed President Franklin D. Roosevelt's Social Security Act, the average life expectancy in America was 60 for males and 64 for females. There was only one Social Security recipient for every seventeen contributors. President Roosevelt envisioned that no individual taxpayer would ever have to pay more than $100 a year into Social Security. Changes in technology, new illnesses, the ratio of recipients to contributors, demographics and an extension of life expectancy to seventy-five years destroyed that prediction.

In 1965, when Congress passed the Medicare and Medicaid acts to create coverage for the elderly and poor, the average life expectancy was 67 for males and 74 for females. But, advances and improvements in health care continued to stretch life expectancies. By 1995, life expectancy is projected to rise to 73 years for males and 80 years for females, with the fastest growing population cohort in the U.S. being the group past age eighty-five. This has affected our ability to fund health care because people over sixty-five years consume four times the health care services of people under sixty-five. People over eighty-five years consume twice as much health care as those between sixty-five and eighty-five. Moreover, their conditions are usually chronic rather than episodic, requiring continuous, sometimes intensive care at greater cost.

Life expectancy at birth and at 65 years

United States: Select Year Estimates 1900-1986 & Projections 1990-2040

Year	At Birth		At 65 Years	
	Male	Female	Male	Female
1900	46.3	48.3	N/A	N/A
1935	59.9	63.9	N/A	N/A
1950	65.6	71.0	12.7	15.0
1965	66.8	73.7	12.9	16.2
1970	67.1	74.8	13.0	16.8
1980	70.1	77.6	14.2	18.4
1985	71.2	78.2	14.6	18.6
1986*	71.5	78.5	14.8	19.0
1990+	72.1	79.0	15.0	19.4
1995+	72.8	79.7	15.4	19.8
2000+	73.5	80.4	15.7	20.3
2010+	74.4	81.3	16.2	21.0
2020+	74.9	81.8	16.6	21.4
2030+	75.4	82.3	17.0	21.8
2040+	75.9	82.8	17.3	22.3

* Provisional data.
+ Projected data.

SOURCE: Bureau of the Census, *Historical Statistics of the United States, Colonial Times to 1970.* Gregory Spencer, *Projections of the Population of the United States by Age, Sex and Race: 1988 to 2080*, Bureau of the Census, U.S. Department of Commerce, P. 25, Number 1018.

Although little can be done to ameliorate these demographic trends, the duplication of resources and advanced technology can be harnessed, if it is properly understood.

HEALTH CARE EVOLUTION

In most industries worldwide, the advancement of high-tech equipment has generally served to bring prices down. This dynamic fails in health care because of the unique evolution of its structure and application of new technology.

Health care began as charity services, run by volunteers in large old houses. These were usually alms houses, where patients went to die. Family doctors, armed primarily with only sulfur for a pain killer, directed most of their treatments at making dying patients comfortable. On occasion they would set bones, remove bullets, or seal wounds, but usually if the patient's immune system did not correct the problem, death or permanent disability followed.

The dawning of modern medicine began near the turn of the century when X-rays were introduced and a new way of diagnosing commenced. The X-rays allowed physicians, for the first time, to look inside the body without being invasive. Hospitals evolved into places where patients could be treated on an episodic basis and cured. Aseptic technique blossomed and matured as targeted and broad-spectrum antibiotics such as penicillin were introduced in the early 1940s.

EXPLOSION OF KNOWLEDGE

By World War II, the development of medical technology and knowledge had begun to accelerate. Synthetic drugs and inoculation solutions gained nationwide usage and felled diseases such as small pox, measles and polio. In the 1960s and 1970s, advancements began exploding exponentially. By the 1980s, medical researchers were learning more about medicine every five years than had been learned in all previous time.

Computers and other technological advancements spawned sophisticated ways of diagnosing conditions, identifying abnormalities and problems, and treating patients. Research on animals and humans produced dramatic breakthroughs in the treatment of cancer and other diseases.

Advancements in other fields, such as aerospace, defense and transportation—also provided health care with thousands of technological applications. One example is the accelerated evolution from X-rays to CT (computerized axial tomography) scanners, MRI (magnetic resonance imaging) capability, and PET (positron emission tomography) technology.

Lasers, fiberoptics, and telecommunications, all developed for other industries, have also yielded tremendous applications to health care. Advancements have come on all fronts for health providers. In the pharmaceutical industry, for example, technological advances used to occur once every twenty-four months. Today, one occurs every twenty-four hours.

PROLIFERATION OF SPECIALISTS

At the end of World War II, Congress turned its attention to America's health. With the Hill-Burton Act in 1946, Congress expressed its wish to place hospitals in every county and doctors in every town. Fifty-nine percent of the Hill-Burton funds went to support community general acute care hospitals. Millions in federal funds were freed to flow into the health care industry and the U.S. Department of Health and Welfare's top priority was to increase the number of doctors. Millions of dollars were spent building and staffing new medical schools and there was even strong sentiment in favor of national health insurance, which ultimately led to the enactment of Medicare and Medicaid.

Hill-Burton expenditure by facility distribution

Expend Distribution Percentage	Facility Type
59%	General Hospitals
19	Public Health Centers
8	Nursing Homes
5	Outpatient Facilities
4	Rehabilitation Facilities
1	T.B. Facilities
1	Mental Health
1	State Health
1	Chronic Disease
1	Community Mental Health Centers
TOTAL: 100%	

SOURCE: Health Care Financing Administration, Public Health Service, Health Resources and Services Administration, Bureau of Health Resources, Division of Facilities Compliance.

By 1950, the role of America's physicians had dramatically changed. While their predecessors had been one-horse family doctors, who were expected to treat everything, including, at times, sick livestock, the post-World War II physicians gained an elevated economic stature and social role. They became gatekeepers of the burgeoning health care system. Although most were paid on a fee-for-service basis, they also played the dual role of patient advocate and provider of patient-care services. It was a problematic arrangement sometimes creating a conflict of interest.

The physician's coveted stature quickly led to a profusion of doctors and other health providers, which in turn led to expansionist competition and jurisdictional disputes. Advancements in technology helped to create specialties—and the pressurized industry quickly spread out horizontally. Fierce turf battles ensued and enfranchisement and licensure efforts intensified.

The number of physicians grew from less than 75,000 in 1940 to 300,000 in 1967, and to more than 600,000 in 1992. Meanwhile, the proliferation in specialties skyrocketed. Twenty-five physician specialties and fifty-six subspecialties now have accredited U.S. training programs. In 1940, fewer than 20 percent of all U.S. physicians were specialists. Today, that number has jumped to more than 60 percent, the highest percentage worldwide.

Doctors in the United States: An unhealthy mix

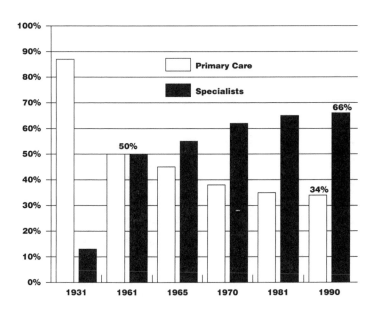

SOURCE: Council on Graduate Medical Education, October 1992.

With each specialist group battling to gain a market niche, the health care system became increasingly stratified and segmented. Jurisdictional disputes became more important than seamless delivery of health care services.

While free-market competition usually drives prices down, among medical providers it seems to operate in an inverse fashion—the more specialists there are, the higher the utilization, and thus costs. Part of the reason for this is that specialization requires long and costly training, much of it supported through government grants and patient-care revenues. The major factors, however, are the higher compensation of specialists, and the consumption of resources and utilization of services, which are fueled by more doctors. The benefit of increased competition was lost in the helter-skelter horizontal expansion of expensive facilities, services, technology, specialties and sub-specialties.

CONVENIENCE-STORE MENTALITY

In part, this costly expansion was fueled by America's own raised expectations. Television helped foster the idea that physicians, like Robert Young's Dr. Welby, could cure almost anything. People began to turn to doctors and medicine more and more to find solutions for their physical and mental problems. The feeling was that a hospital should be like a 24-hour convenience store, but with the latest technology and breakthroughs. As a result, most urban areas in the U.S. now boast more high-tech medical wizardry than many countries around the world. Several metropolitan communities, for example, have more cardiac surgery units and MRI scanners than all of Canada. The number of hospital beds in the U.S. soared to meet demands generated by Medicare and Medicaid. Racing to fulfill the public policy mandate and public demand, individual health care providers answered the call with more facilities, services, technology and resources. The new order changed every aspect of health care, creating considerable challenges. Meeting today's needs in an affordable manner and with contemporary sophistication has become our nemesis.

Hospitals and beds
United States: Select Years 1957-1991

Year	Hospitals	Annual % Change	Beds	Annual % Change
1957	5,309	-	594,529	-
1960	5,407	0.8%	639,057	3.1%
1965	5,736	0.4	741,292	2.8
1970	5,859	0.1	848,232	2.7
1975*	5,875	0.0	941,844	1.7
1980	5,830	-0.2	988,387	0.5
1985	5,732	-0.5	1,000,678	1.6
1986	5,678	-0.9	978,375	-2.3
1987	5,611	-1.2	958,312	-2.1
1988	5,533	-1.4	946,038	-1.3
1989	5,455	-1.4	933,318	-1.3
1990	5,384	-1.3	927,360	-0.6
1991	5,342	-0.8	924,049	-0.4

* Prior to 1972, data relate to the term "short-term general and other special" hospitals. Since 1972, data relate to the category "community hospitals" which excludes units of institutions that are included in the 1957-1970 data.

SOURCE: American Hospital Association, *Hospitals Guide Issue*, 1957-1970, Chicago. American Hospital Association, *Hospital Statistics*, 1975-1992, Chicago.

Hospitals responded to the call for more beds, technology and services. From 1965 to 1975, the number of beds increased 35 percent. By 1985, the peak of 1 million hospital beds was reached. The national evolution of reforms started a downturn in beds that is accelerating each year. By 1992, the United States had less than 900,000 hospital beds.

MASKING THE PAIN

The growth of third-party payer insurance and governmental programs masked the pain of rising costs. Health insurance first became a part of mainstream America in 1960, when the steel industry employees negotiated health care coverage into their labor contracts. In 1964, the United Automobile Workers followed suit and health insurance soon became an automatic benefit in most intermediate-sized and large corporations. The insurance was inexpensive and federal tax laws encouraged its acceptance by allowing employers to fully deduct its cost and by declaring the benefits as nontaxable income for individuals.

At first, the design worked well. More people than ever had accessible health care and the health care industry was making great strides in quality improvement. But from 1950 to 1992, the percent of health care expenses actually paid by individuals dropped from 65 percent to 20 percent. Since individuals paid only twenty cents for every dollar of health care they consumed, they became isolated from the real costs. Meanwhile, the exemption of employer-paid insurance premiums from state and federal income tax grew to an annual subsidy for providers and payers of almost $60 billion in 1992. This served to further insulate the American public from the true cost of health care. Eventually, as insurance companies usurped the role of legal watchdog over health care prices, the final bond between consumers and the cost of the health care was cut.

Today individuals are typically unaware of hospital or physician charges, relying on insurance to take care of them. The result of such insensitivity has been excess demand, system abuse, and, finally, the society's expectation that health care is a right, regardless of an individual's ability to pay for it. The truth is that every American bears the costs, through higher health care bills and taxes, increased product prices, or through inaccessibility to health services.

THE MEDICAID SHELL GAME

The United States has not benefitted from a consistent governmental policy on health care. In fact, the government's message has been almost arbitrary, changing seasonally with the political tides, with no overall long-term vision, direction or focus.

All of us are responsible. But the federal government must bear the primary blame. Federal policy has consistently widened the gap between demand and available resources. Rather than providing solutions, governmental policies have caused many of the problems.

Medicaid, which cost more than $121 billion in state and federal funds in 1992, is failing. Costs are rising at more than 12 percent annually. Only 38 percent of the poor were eligible in 1992, compared with 76 percent in 1965 when Medicaid was created.

While payments differ from state to state, the average Medicaid payment to hospitals covers only 82 percent of the actual cost.

The government's ineffective cost-containment efforts have floundered. Medicaid costs continue to grow faster than almost any other governmental program. In 1983, Congress passed the Medicare Prospective Payment System (PPS), as a cost-saving program. The PPS pays hospitals a fixed amount for each inpatient diagnosis, regardless of how long the patient stays. While the Medicare

PPS shortened hospital stays, it also increased nursing home admissions, largely paid through Medicaid. Now, nearly 70 percent of the Medicaid budget is consumed by the elderly, blind, and disabled, while millions of economically disadvantaged people have no coverage.

Cost shifts – Overall gains and losses by payer
United States – 1991

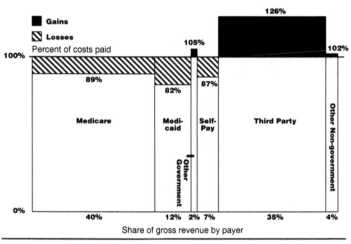

SOURCE: 1991 AHA Annual Survey.

The recession of the early 1990s has had a major impact on Medicaid caseloads and Medicaid expenditures have risen. As the federal government attempted to limit its Medicaid matching payments, states experimented with two strategies to make ends meet. The first was to obtain more federal Medicaid matching funds through voluntary contributions, provider taxes, and inter-governmental transfers. The second was the attempt to transfer health care obligations to local governments and private payers. These off-loading actions were more pronounced in states where local governments own and operate safety-net hospitals.

The recession and the Medicaid shell game have produced an unparalleled period of destabilization. Cost containment has degenerated into arbitrary cuts in payments to providers, eligibility, and benefits.

MEDICARE SHIFTING COSTS

Medicare has fared little better. The program now pays for only 89 percent of the cost of treating its hospital patients, leaving the remaining expenses to be shifted to private patients and their insurance companies.

Health providers have been forced to shift an increasing financial burden to the insurance carriers by continuously raising their prices. The carriers, in turn, pass the price hikes on to customers through increased premiums, locking out millions of people who can no longer afford coverage. This "cost shift" is a hidden tax that government is willing to impose but reluctant to acknowledge.

Private industry, however, is well aware of the damage done by such cost shifts. General Motor's O'Brien points out that as health care costs grab an increasing percentage of the gross domestic product, non-health care jobs in the private sector will be lost. O'Brien projects that up to 120,000 jobs in the automobile industry alone will disappear by the year 2000 due to increased health care costs.

Some employers' response to this pressure is to limit the number of people covered by their plans by expanding temporary, part-time, and contract employees, who are ineligible for employer-paid health benefits. Another response is to require employees to pay a larger share of health care costs.

BEHAVIORAL CHANGES

The evolution of health care in America has produced several behavioral patterns that must be changed. For example, health care providers are motivated to concentrate on curative rather than preventative methods and advancements.

Much rhetoric is heard in support of preventative medicine, wellness promotion, and stopping the "do-more-get-more" race. But the public's demand for unrestricted choice of physicians, and unwillingness to pay out-of-pocket deductibles and co-payments keep the roadblocks to progress in place.

At the same time, the insulation that third-party payers provide has sapped the consumer's incentive to engage in good health practices by taking responsibility for their decisions. Unfortunately, we too often ignore the consequences of poor health habits and behavior patterns detrimental to ourselves and others. Abuse of tobacco, drugs, and alcohol; violence; and other destructive lifestyle behaviors have a direct correlation to increased health care costs.

A case of child abuse, which culminates in the emergency room, is a common example of this. Jason was a three-year-old, who was physically abused by his father. The family had no health insurance. One evening, his father beat him so severely that he suffered a broken rib, which also punctured a lung. When Jason arrived at the hospital, he appeared lethargic and complained that his chest and head hurt. The doctor on duty immediately ran a CT scan, to see if a head injury had occurred, and ordered X-rays. Because they suspected child abuse, the doctor had a complete series of X-rays done so he could look for bones that might be in various stages of healing—a sure sign a history of child abuse exists.

The CT scan came back clear, but the X-rays showed a broken rib and collapsed lung. To treat the lung, the doctor admitted Jason for three days so a chest tube could be inserted and his lung reinflated. When Jason was released, he had incurred a substantial bill that his family would most likely never pay.

Similarly, thousands of patients were treated in hospitals during the 1992 Los Angeles riots. Most were victims of personal aggression. Hospital emergency rooms were inundated with victims attacked in their places of business or homes. Los Angeles-area hospitals lost more than $10 million treating people injured during the riots, while businesses lost hundreds of millions of dollars due to the violence.

While poor health habits and dangerous behavioral patterns have become prevalent, government policies have also created a scenario whereby providers are rewarded monetarily for providing more and more services and insurance carriers, as intermediaries, seek greater profits through the collection of more premiums. Moreover, they have instituted regressive post-care auditing of bills, utilization reviews, and other activities designed to limit their payments. Working simultaneously to cut risks at the other end, carriers have expanded exclusionary rules, some even to the point of using genetic studies to assess potential health risks. The result is that an increasing number of people are excluded from insurance coverage.

THE HEALTH CARE SOLUTION

This book contains a plan that re-aligns the incentives of health providers, patients, payers, and government, so that common goals and a common vision can be established. Changes in attitudes, understandings, and behaviors will hopefully follow. A new set of positive personal incentives for providers is created, based on competitive collaboration and market forces, rather than governmental attempts to change behavior through negative incentives, such as fines, regulations, controls, or restrictions.

The primary goal is to build a system that provides quality, affordable health care for all Americans. Moreover, some of the secondary benefits of the new paradigm are significant within themselves. For example, the worker's compensation dilemma, with its incumbent, legal red tape and financial problems, should be eliminated with respect to health care. It should not matter when or how you are injured. Accomplishing this alone would be worth the change, but it is only one of many goals of the new paradigm. Other benefits include the elimination of the $1.25 billion annual cost of hospital audits and utilization reviews conducted by insurance companies; a new emphasis on illness prevention by providers; a reduction in unnecessary surgeries and other procedures; and fewer institutional beds. Rebuilding the system, though, will require vision and extraordinary leadership from government and health care providers. Physicians must be motivated to see beyond their current focus on jurisdictional disputes and specialty enfranchisements. Hospitals must become effective cost centers rather than generators of revenue. The health care system itself must move beyond the myriad uncoordinated services and specialties, which belie seamless health care.

America began with a primitive form of health care and developed the most sophisticated, but most expensive, system in the world. Now, we need to retool and chart a new course that continues the momentum created by the remarkable technological and service breakthroughs, to bring them into line with the country's financial means.

Policy makers must forge ahead and make the hard choices that will create the proper balance among all interests. Specifically, employers and employees must have a system compatible with their interests as well as those of the health providers.

Accomplishing this requires a fundamental restructuring of the way health care is funded and delivered.

COMPETITION
GONE AWRY

In the years following World War II, America rose to a preeminent economic position in world affairs, boasting the most competitive marketplace on earth. Free enterprise was recognized as the most successful form of commerce and competition was seen as the vital force driving product innovation, quality, and price. If a company was not efficient enough to provide a low-price, high-quality product, it fell by the wayside, beaten by those that could.

That belief was underscored by the economic failures and withering of human ingenuity in the Soviet Union and other countries that prohibited or restricted free competition. In general, Americans came to trust the dynamics of the free marketplace to protect against economic stagnation, high prices, and inferior goods and services. Perhaps that is why the failures of the highly competitive health care system came as such a surprise.

It was assumed by government leaders and others that health care, like America's other industries, would thrive within a free-market environment. Providers would be forced to keep prices down in order to compete. Quality service would be almost guaranteed.

By the 1980s, though, it became painfully clear that health care did not respond to market forces with lower prices or costs. Rather than stimulate efficient operation and low prices, competition caused the opposite. The result was duplicated resources and excess capacity, unneeded services, over-utilization, and rising prices. The Institute of Medicine has estimated that the use of new technologies and overuse of existing capacity account for as much as 50 percent of the annual increase in health care costs.

At the same time, specialists dominated the system, placing an emphasis on end-stage intervention and high-cost utilization. Increasingly, people entered the system at its most expensive points—the specialist's door and the hospital emergency department. Emphasis was placed on the costly catastrophic side of the health care equation.

The results were predictable—health costs are rising at double the rate of national inflation, nearly 75 million people are underinsured or not insured at all, and parts of the system are edging toward the brink of economic collapse. Yet, while the effects of the failures are apparent, the reasons are not. Despite rhetoric to the contrary, there is no quick fix, no simple solution to be legislated and implemented overnight. The problems lie deeply rooted within society and the structure of the system itself. Nothing less than universal systemic reform will bring health care into balance.

DIFFERENT RULES

Fundamental to understanding the problems within the health care system is the recognition that it differs from virtually every other industry. On one hand, it is considered by most Americans to be a right and a cornerstone of "the public good," much like education. Yet, while education is publicly financed and a guaranteed right through age sixteen, health care is only partially funded and no rights are affirmed.

THE GUISE OF QUALITY

The troubling result of government shunning its responsibilities has been that providers, fearful of losing their revenue base, attempt to stay a step ahead by providing an increasing array of technology and services. More tests and surgeries are performed, more outpatients are treated, and a greater assortment of diagnostic and therapeutic services are administered than ever before. Every institution, every group practice, and nearly every individual practitioner attempts to provide as many services as possible. Many providers have been incentivized to believe the best way to prosper is to promote the services themselves, maximize the utilization of technology, and receive more for doing more.

Community hospital inpatient and outpatient surgical operations

United States: Select Years 1972-1991

	Surgical Operations				Inpatient Surgeries		Outpatient Surgeries	
Year	Total	Annual % change	/1000 pop.	to Admissions	Total	/1000 pop.	Total	/1000 pop.
1972	14,768,063	..	70.6	.48%	NA	..	NA	..
1975	16,663,846	2.9%	78.0	.50	NA	..	NA	..
1980	18,767,666	2.7	83.2	.52	NA	..	NA	..
1982	19,593,639	1.9	85.2	.54	15,532,578	67.5%	4,061,061	17.7%
1983	19,844,908	1.3	85.5	.55	15,130,404	65.2	4,714,504	20.3
1984	19,908,241	0.3	85.0	.57	14,378,580	61.4	5,529,661	23.6
1985	20,113,350	1.0	85.1	.60	13,161,991	55.7	6,951,359	29.4
1986	20,469,134	1.8	85.9	.63	12,222,472	51.3	8,246,662	34.6
1987	20,817,629	1.7	86.5	.66	11,691,432	48.6	9,126,197	37.9
1988	21,411,138	2.8	88.1	.68	11,383,578	47.3	10,027,560	41.3
1989	21,340,280	-2.9	87.1	.69	10,989,409	44.8	10,350,871	42.2
1990	21,914,868	2.7	88.5	.70	10,844,916	43.8	11,069,952	44.7
1991	22,405,051	2.2	89.4	.72	10,693,243	42.7	11,711,808	46.7

SOURCE: American Hospital Association, *Annual Hospital Survey, 1972-1992*, Chicago.

Today, unnecessary medical procedures cost American consumers nearly $130 billion annually— 20 percent of the entire health care budget, according to the Consumer's Union, an organization based in Washington, DC, that represents consumers' interests. Cesarean sections, hysterectomies, some coronary bypasses, magnetic resonance imaging and other imaging services, laboratory procedures, and diagnostic tests are among the most overused procedures. It is clear that while health care professionals carve out pieces of new turf under the guise of access and quality, one of the main motivators is financial in nature.

Physicians began investing in laboratories, radiology and imaging services, ambulatory surgical services, post-surgical recovery facilities, and many other diagnostic and therapeutic services to which they refer patients or provide the services directly. (This practice is limited under Medicare and is illegal in some states.) Typically, the cost of providing these services is high because they require the newest line of technological diagnostic and treatment tools. Investors must receive a financial return on these investments, creating an ever-expanding incentive to order more tests, procedures, and services. When this happens, when services are rendered to pay for capital outlays as opposed to necessary care, it's clear the system has taken a turn in the wrong direction.

THE ABSURD DECEPTION

In response to the cost shifts and escalating prices, insurance carriers have tried to control costs in several ways, including a variety of discounted care and managed care arrangements. These include exclusive- and preferred-provider agreements, specialty-provider contract arrangements, fee schedules, and other individual discount contracts. The situation has become so absurd that very few third-party payers pay "retail" for health care.

Most third-party payer contracts with hospitals and physicians rely on discounts and other adjustments, which means that with virtually no one paying the retail value of the bills, charges have to be greatly inflated. This trend was started primarily by government's underpayments.

For a hospital to receive $1 in net revenue, it must charge an increase of at least $4 on the bills it sends out. As a result, the real cost of health care becomes even more difficult to identify. Costs are shifted, and billing charges are arranged to maximize revenues in a shrinking universe of bill-paying payers. It has become a deceptive, high-stakes game of contracting, with each side struggling to stay one step ahead of the other.

What has gone unrecognized in this locked battle, is that neither side can ultimately win because the model itself is defective. The incentives and goals, inherently misaligned within the system, have doomed both sides.

HOSPITALS FACE A GRIM FUTURE

A major casualty of the crisis has been America's hospitals. The majority are experiencing negative patient revenue margins, even though the average hospital bill has nearly tripled in the past ten years.

Community hospital patient margin and total expenses
United States: 1980-1991 (000)

Year	Patient Margin	Community Hospital Expenses	Expense Annual % Increase
1980	N/A	$ 76,851,146	16.4%
1981	N/A	90,572,422	17.9
1982	-3.0%	104,875,624	15.8
1983	-2.6	116,437,675	11.0
1984	-1.7	123,336,420	5.9
1985	-0.6	130,499,066	5.8
1986	-2.0	140,654,175	7.8
1987	-3.6	152,584,542	8.4
1988	-4.7	168,557,191	10.5
1989	-4.5	184,897,504	9.7
1990	-4.2	203,692,591	10.2
1991	-3.6	225,023,388	10.5

SOURCE: American Hospital Association, Selected Hospital Statistics, 1982-1991, "A Statistical Profile," Chicago, 1992.

American Hospital Association, *Hospital Statistics*, Chicago, 1976-1992.

A large part of the problem is that for ethical and legal reasons, hospitals must continue to treat the millions of Americans who cannot pay their bills. Thus, hospitals are forced to absorb more than $20 billion annually in unpaid bills, which does not include the billions in shortfalls created by Medicare and Medicaid. Moreover, hospital workers' wages have soared in recent years in connection with the need for highly skilled technicians to operate the increasing amount of high-tech equipment.

Community hospital bad debt and charity expenses
United States: 1982-1991 (000)

Year	Bad Debt	Charity	Bad Debt And Charity	Annual % Change
1982	$ 4,544,273	$1,989,498	$ 6,533,771	---
1983	5,485,310	2,351,438	7,836,748	19.94%
1984	6,981,753	2,556,592	9,538,345	21.71
1985	7,040,846	2,485,387	9,526,233	-0.13
1986	7,829,117	3,834,327	11,663,444	22.44
1987	8,565,584	4,075,853	12,641,437	8.39
1988	9,650,317	4,531,855	14,182,172	12.19
1989	11,192,939	4,446,173	15,639,112	10.27
1990	11,572,782	6,218,540	17,791,322	13.76
1991	13,151,799	7,321,538	20,473,337	15.07

SOURCE: American Hospital Association, *Selected Hospital Statistics 1982-1991*, "A Statistical Profile," Chicago, 1992.

With increasing services offered through outpatient and physicians' office facilities, hospital usage dropped drastically in the past decade. There are nearly 200,000 excess hospital beds nationwide, which directly and indirectly costs more than $3 billion annually. Estimates suggest that more than one-third of U.S. hospitals will be closed or used for alternative purposes by the year 2000.

Community hospital outpatient visits and inpatient admissions and patient days

United States: Select Years 1975-1991 (000)

	OUTPATIENT			INPATIENT			
Year	Visits	Annual % Change	Visits /1,000 Pop.	Admissions	Admission /1,000 Pop.	Patient Days	Patient Days /1,000 Pop.
1975	190,672	0.9	892	33,435	156	257,594	1,205
1980	202,310	1.8	896	36,143	160	273,085	1,210
1985	218,716	3.2	926	33,449	142	236,619	1,002
1986	231,912	6.0	973	32,378	136	229,448	962
1987	245,524	5.9	1,021	31,601	131	227,015	944
1988	269,044	9.6	1,108	31,429	129	226,688	933
1989	285,712	6.2	1,166	31,116	127	225,437	920
1990	301,329	5.5	1,216	31,181	126	225,972	912
1991	322,048	6.9	1,285	31,064	124	222,858	889

SOURCE: American Hospital Association, *Hospital Statistics*, 1975-1992, Chicago.

CONSUMER STRESS

Consumers are another major factor driving up costs. Insurance—whether it is Medicare, Medicaid, employer-covered, or individually paid premiums—has isolated us from the real costs of health care. Thus, consumer decisions are not made under the same circumstances as they are for other free-market items and services. Typically, if a service costs more than consumers are willing to pay, the service is refused or an alternative is found. This dynamic doesn't hold true, however, when we don't know or care about the real cost of that service. This insurance buffer keeps consumers from paying the real costs of life-style choices that adversely affect health. For example, smokers cost the nation more than $52 billion annually in health expenses and lost productivity. Diagnosis, treatment, and drug abuse-related costs add up to more than $3 billion. More than 2.5 million people are victims of violent injury each year, costing a billion dollars more in treatment and court costs.

To complicate the situation, individuals are generally in a mental or physical state of stress when they need health care. Conversely, when consumers go to purchase a house, automobile, food, clothes, or other products, they are usually in a position to shop and carefully weigh their options. They have the time and opportunity to evaluate and choose, balancing the factors of economics: convenience, quality, service, price, and style. However, when people need health care in most cases, price is not heavily weighed—regardless of whether patients are adequately covered. Health care transcends other services in immediate personal importance and thus does not follow our free-market, cost-analysis methods. In effect, we have no real gauge to judge how much health care is worth.

The fact remains that people expect high-level health care when they require it, usually without regard to cost. The government, in an attempt to comply with this expectation and manage costs at the same time, has enacted a number of laws, some of which, unfortunately, have made the situation worse.

MISSING THE MARK

Some consumer-protection legislation has also had negative side effects. Federal and state laws require that hospitals treat every patient presented at the emergency room—the most expensive point of entry. Providers, who are severely penalized for noncompliance, must treat all patients whether or not the situation actually calls for emergency intervention. Other laws and regulations require that patient transfers be made only under specifically defined circumstances, which include approval of the patient. This often results in patients remaining in high-cost treatment areas, when they could safely be transferred or referred to lower cost alternatives.

Since 1984, Congress has made more than fifteen adjustments in the Medicare DRG Hospital Prospective Payment System, primarily because so many inequities exist. Yet, none of these "quick fixes" have repaired the system, partly because Prospective Payment System applies only to hospitals. Compatible policies affecting patients, physicians, and other providers have not been enacted.

Several U.S. Department of Health and Human Services (DHHS) actions are illustrative. In an attempt to limit and redistribute payments among physicians, a resource-based, relative value scale (RBRVS) payment system was unveiled in 1992. By simply cutting payments and shifting funds among physicians, DHHS proposed to save money and improve access. In reality, the rule has penalized many doctors and induced many more physicians to peel off and carve out hospital services to preserve their traditional income levels. This perpetuates the negative spiral of unnecessary duplication of services, adds costs, and fragments care.

Another rule that misses the mark is the Medicare/Medicaid Fraud and Abuse Safe Harbors, promulgated as a haven for joint ventures and self-referrals. The 40 percent ownership and 40 percent revenue limits have caused fragmentation and higher costs, and have reduced coordinated provider influence over utilization of services. By combining hospitals and physicians within the 40 percent limits, the federal government dug a new bottomless pit. The door for 60 percent independent investors is wide open. Private middle-layer investors are marching in with 60 percent financing and control. The pie pan is stretched horizontally and a new set of nonproviders brought to the table to dine. The demand for investment return translates into more technology, facilities, and services. The final result is higher utilization, and thus costs, with no improvement in quality.

STATES FALTER

States, meanwhile, are trying to control their growing Medicaid expenditures through a wide range of initiatives, most of which are no more imaginative than restricting access or shifting costs. Methods include restricting eligibility, benefits, and payments; selective contracting; retroactive denials; and complicated treatment authorization and payment rules. Local governments are being asked to shoulder increasing costs and short-sighted "managed care" permutations are being imposed. Rather than create realistic and congruent incentives, partial solutions are devised. Most of them foster fraud, abuse, restricted access, or decreased quality.

Squeezed by these well-meaning, but misguided efforts, insurers are scrambling to protect their interests by limiting options, engaging in predatory practices, and negotiating increasingly restrictive payment arrangements with providers. The ultimate results are reduced access, higher costs, wider gaps among stakeholders, and the restriction of needed services and facilities.

NO HALFWAY SOLUTIONS

In 1992 alone, some seventy different legislative health reform proposals were introduced in Congress, though none have been enacted. They vary in many specifics, but most fall generally into one of four categories:

- The employer-sponsored plan seeks to achieve universal access by building on the present system of employer-based coverage with government covering the indigent, unemployed, and elderly.
- The "Play-or-Pay" proposal gives employers the option to provide private coverage or be taxed so that the employee is covered by the government rather than by employer-secured insurance.
- The government-payer approach, most likened to the British or Canadian national health care systems, makes government the payer for defined health coverage. Financing would come from payroll, income taxes, other taxes, or combinations of them.
- The incremental approach is based on voluntary expansion of coverage through incentives and reforms in various areas which influence health care, such as insurance.

While these proposals have merit, they are temporary solutions at best. At worst, they lead us toward government control because they fail to strike at the heart of the problem.

THE NEW MODEL

No amount of mere tinkering will achieve the goal we must reach—affordable, universal access to a uniform benefit package characterized by high-quality care. Only a reconstructed model, based on balanced incentives and managed collaboration, a coordinated payment system, and a carefully constructed delivery mechanism, will provide the ingredients crucial to long-term success.

A number of elements must be included in the new model. The plan must change provider incentives to reduce technological and service duplication, while encouraging efficient resource allocation and utilization, joint decision making, and high- quality care. Accountability must become a personal reality.

Incentives for private carriers must also be changed. Rather than competing for the low-risk, healthy patients, insurance companies and others must be given the motivation to compete for all residents, regardless of age, race, occupation, or health status.

It will take effort, patience, and a clear vision to achieve these goals. But, the public desire for affordable, accessible health care has never been stronger. A recent nationwide Gallup poll indicated that 89 percent of the public supports serious health care reform. The administration's efforts to develop a national health care policy has been page-one news throughout most of 1993. More than ever before, Americans are gravely concerned about the future of health care—and for good reason.

Lack of health care coverage is not limited to a single economic group. In fact, the fastest-growing segments of uninsured are those whose income is between $25,000 and $50,000. Escalating health care costs, skyrocketing workers' compensation costs, changes in social policy and a persistent recession threaten to undercut the entire economy. Moreover, these forces have become a psychological burden to many Americans. Those without coverage often suffer stress from the knowledge that they are without insurance. Others, who have employer-provided coverage, fear losing their insurance as much as they fear losing their jobs. Another Gallup Poll in California revealed that nearly one-third of all workers remain job-locked because they are afraid they'll lose their coverage if they change employment.

PRECEDENT TO CHANGE

Adapting to changing times is scarcely a new idea. The aerospace, transportation, automobile, electronics, and defense industries are all undergoing restructuring to meet emerging public priorities and the challenges of new competition. Successful companies and organizations realize that to survive, they must remain flexible and adapt to change. This includes a constant redefinition of roles and systemic procedures.

It is vital to recognize that there is no validity to the argument that health care cannot change because it is tradition-bound, or that providers have an inherent right to play their present roles in the future. In fact, to be successful the new system or model cannot preserve all the stakeholders' roles that have evolved during the past fifty years.

MANAGED COLLABORATION

The new paradigm will require the acceptance of some intriguing ideas. Choice, quality, service, and price can all be blended into the model if the underlying differences between health care and other parts of the economy and society are recognized.

Managed collaboration will produce the desired results of high-quality, low-price services, if there is a level playing field where players can compete evenly and consumers have the power to make wise choices and purchases.

ALTERNATIVE SOLUTIONS

As the U.S. health care system wobbles and sways under the burden of rising costs and payment strangulation, the systems in other industrialized countries are coming under increased scrutiny. Ironically, many foreign countries are looking at alternative solutions which are based on aspects of the U.S. system.

Because health systems typically reflect the social, economic, and political values of a given country, analyzing other nations' systems is not an easy task. What is acceptable in one country may be abhorrent in another. Moreover, few modern systems are the result of carefully designed plans; they are the result of political struggles, social expectations, and the power of interest groups within the country. Most are built through a collection of subsequent reforms, mirroring the desires of the political factions in power at that time.

Yet, in reviewing the differing systems worldwide, one commonality emerges. Although they vary in specifics, nearly every system outside the U.S. has a common component—some form of budgetary predictability. In one way or another, whether through financing, delivery, utilization, regulation of resources, or a combination of these, most other countries have opted for government to play a role in containing costs.

GOVERNMENTAL CONTROL

At one end of the spectrum are the socialized systems of Scandinavia and Great Britain, where the government provides the facilities, trains physicians and other practitioners, and pays for the services rendered. Most providers in these countries are paid on a salary or agreed budgetary basis, rather than the traditional fee-for-service basis prevalent in the U.S. and several other countries.

At the other end of the spectrum are countries like Germany, New Zealand, and Japan, which employ both the private and public sectors. The U.S. system also includes both private and public financing, but there is one fundamental difference. Unlike most other countries, the U.S. does not utilize some form of overall budgetary predictability. The fact that the U.S. operates under completely different values and economic dynamics must be taken into account when evaluating whether we can "borrow" other systems.

In England, for example, the National Health Service is operated at the federal level with regional directors responsible for monies paid to hospitals and other providers. The system is tax-financed and generally free at the point of delivery. General practitioners act as gatekeepers and determine which services are provided and when referrals occur. Most family practice physicians do not have privileges at hospitals, but must refer patients when hospital care is needed.

Because the federal government limits technology expenditures and services from the top down, a queuing (waiting list) system exists. Facilities are limited, usually old, and are utilized to the maximum. Top-down budgetary limits usually have resulted in less than state-of-the-art technology, services and professionals. This strict governmental control has had both positive and negative effects.

Although some of the reporting standards differ and other components of the comparisons may not be identical, the following charts give an indication that the resources devoted to health care in the United States outpace all other nations.

The queuing system in some countries has become so choked that there are often lengthy waits for some services, while others are simply unavailable. Moreover, health care is often administered in a dreary atmosphere where patients are given over to the discipline of the queue. Meanwhile, chronic underfunding has limited the services and resources, and an increasing number of patients receive only inexpensive care. This type of supply control from the top, called implicit rationing, creates a

Total health expenditures as a percentage of GDP*

Twenty-four Countries: Select Years 1960-1991

Country	1960	1965	1970	1975	1980	1985	1988	1989	1990	1991
Australia	4.6%	4.9%	5.0%	5.7%	6.5%	7.7%	7.7%	7.8%	8.2%	8.6%
Austria	4.6	5.0	5.4	7.3	7.9	8.1	8.4	8.4	8.3	8.4
Belgium	3.4	3.9	4.0	5.8	6.6	7.4	7.7	7.6	7.6	7.9
Canada†	5.5	6.1	7.2	7.3	7.4	8.5	8.8	9.0	9.5	10.0
Denmark	3.6	4.8	6.1	6.5	6.8	6.3	6.5	6.5	6.3	6.5
Finland	3.9	4.9	5.7	6.3	6.5	7.2	7.2	7.2	7.8	8.9
France	4.2	5.2	5.8	6.8	7.6	8.5	8.6	8.7	8.8	9.1
Germany	4.7	5.1	5.5	7.8	7.9	8.7	8.8	8.3	8.3	8.5
Greece	3.2	3.6	4.0	4.1	4.3	4.9	5.0	5.4	5.4	5.2
Iceland	1.2	2.8	4.3	5.9	6.4	7.1	8.6	8.6	8.3	8.4
Ireland	4.0	4.4	5.6	7.7	8.5	8.2	7.3	6.9	7.0	7.3
Italy	3.3	4.0	4.8	5.8	6.8	7.0	7.6	7.6	8.1	8.3
Japan	2.9	4.3	4.4	5.5	6.4	6.5	6.6	6.6	6.7	6.8
Luxembourg	-	-	4.1	5.7	6.8	6.8	7.2	6.9	7.2	7.2
Netherlands	3.9	4.4	6.0	7.7	8.2	8.0	8.2	8.1	8.2	8.3
New Zealand	4.4	4.5	5.1	6.4	7.2	6.5	7.1	7.2	7.3	7.6
Norway	3.3	3.9	5.0	6.7	6.6	6.4	7.7	7.4	7.4	7.6
Portugal	-	-	-	6.4	5.9	7.0	7.1	7.2	6.7	6.8
Spain	2.3	2.7	4.1	5.1	5.9	5.7	6.0	6.3	6.6	6.7
Sweden	4.7	5.6	7.2	8.0	9.5	8.8	8.6	8.6	8.6	8.6
Switzerland	3.3	3.8	5.2	7.0	7.3	7.6	7.8	7.5	7.8	7.9
Turkey ‡	-	-	-	-	-	2.8	3.8	3.9	4.0	4.0
United Kingdom	3.9	4.1	4.5	5.5	5.8	6.0	6.1	6.1	6.2	6.6
United States	5.2	6.0	7.4	8.4	9.2	10.5	11.1	11.5	12.2	13.2
AVERAGE	**3.8**	**4.5**	**5.3**	**6.5**	**7.0**	**7.2**	**7.5**	**7.5**	**7.6**	**7.9**

* Includes long term care expenditures.

† Health and Welfare in Canada uses a slightly different definition of Gross Domestic Product (GDP) than is used in GDP figures reported to the OECD.

‡ Average excluding Turkey 1960-1980.

SOURCE: George J. Schieber et al, *Health Affairs*, "International Health Care Expenditure Trends: 1987," fall 1989, Project HOPE, Bethesda. George J. Schieber et al, *Health Affairs*, "Data Watch: "Health Spending, Delivery and Outcomes in OECD Countries," summer, 1993, Project HOPE, Bethesda.

growing equity gap in the system as those rich enough to afford it often seek services outside of the system or even in another country. Increasingly, they look to the U.S. for diagnostic or therapeutic care, because it is available here at almost a moment's notice.

International per capita health spending*

United States Dollars: 1985–1991

Country	Per Capita Health Spending						
	1985	1986	1987	1988	1989	1990	1991
Australia	$ 998	$1,072	$1,112	$1,171	$1,225	$1,310	$1,407
Austria	984	1,046	1,109	1,191	1,298	1,383	1,448
Belgium	879	931	992	1,081	1,153	1,242	1,377
Canada	1,244	1,364	1,461	1,558	1,666	1,811	1,915
Denmark	807	818	890	972	1,013	1,051	1,151
Finland	855	911	979	1,044	1,147	1,291	1,426
France	1,083	1,135	1,193	1,295	1,415	1,528	1,650
Germany	1,175	1,215	1,287	1,409	1,412	1,522	1,659
Greece	282	323	321	334	384	400	404
Iceland	889	1,073	1,220	1,331	1,373	1,379	1,447
Ireland	572	580	596	620	651	748	845
Italy	814	849	955	1,058	1,150	1,296	1,408
Japan	792	839	916	992	1,092	1,119	1,307
Luxembourg	930	978	1,135	1,219	1,267	1,392	1,494
Netherlands	931	990	1,046	1,101	1,176	1,286	1,360
New Zealand	747	806	871	900	954	995	1,047
Norway	846	1,066	1,043	1,112	1,128	1,193	1,305
Portugal	398	389	434	493	548	554	624
Spain	452	472	522	598	682	774	848
Sweden	1,150	1,165	1,240	1,303	1,390	1,455	1,443
Switzerland	1,224	1,267	1,332	1,435	1,498	1,640	1,713
Turkey	66	89	100	110	118	133	142
United States	1,711	1,824	1,962	2,146	2,362	2,601	2,868
United Kingdom ..	685	739	795	858	912	985	1,043
AVERAGE	**$ 855**	**$ 914**	**$ 980**	**$1,055**	**$1,126**	**$1,212**	**$1,305**

* Includes long term health care data.

SOURCE:Organization for Economic Cooperation and Development, *OECD Health Systems: Facts and Trends*, Paris, 1993. National Health Care Expenditures 1991, *Health Care Financing Review*, S. Letsch et al., winter, 1992.

In Germany, a regional system has been established for the delivery of health care services. Private insurers are used, but the insuring companies must comply with federal standards, pay for services, and enroll people irrespective of their financial or health conditions.

Budgets are established at national and regional levels and enforced through negotiations between providers and sick pools administered by third-party carriers. Most physicians are paid on a fee-for-service basis.

In three important ways, the German system shares similarities with those of France, Japan, and the United States. First, medical care is provided by private physicians and by both private and public hospitals. Patients are relatively free to choose their own physicians. Second, the majority of people receive their health insurance coverage through their workplace. Finally, the insurance is provided through multiple third-party insurers.

There is, however, one important difference between health care in these countries and in the U.S. While all three have been able to achieve nearly universal coverage under their systems, the U.S. has not. The reason, once again, is governmental control. The U.S. government concentrates on regulatory standards and underpayments. In Germany, Japan, and France, the respective governments require universal health care coverage, standardize reimbursement policies for most physicians and hospitals, and base insurance rates on total population costs, not on each individual group's expected costs of care.

Such a victory does not come without its own price tag. Increasingly, these countries, and most others opting for strong governmental regulations, are struggling with diminishing incentives for innovation, queuing systems, and rising costs. Recently, fraud and abuse, litigation and a host of other problems have emerged. These challenges point out the difficulty of getting a handle on the continually moving target of health and health care.

THE CANADIAN SYSTEM

The Canadian system, which is often held up as a potential model for the U.S., is struggling with the very problems just mentioned. Canada's publicly funded system is actually made up of different provincial plans that share common features. A public agency in each province makes all payments to providers and hospitals, giving the agency financing and political control.

In 1974, when the program was initiated, the federal government played a much larger role, paying for 60 percent of the health care system. Today, it pays for only 40 percent, having shifted the cost to the provinces.

Canada operates a single-collector program, in which the government collects and houses all funds. The program was originally funded through tax revenues, but now some provinces impose payroll taxes on employers to supplement financing of services. The provincial governments determine overall increases in hospital budgets and physician fees and regulate the acquisition of resources, including equipment and services.

In a major departure from the U.S. system, Canadian physicians are precluded from offering, or investing in, technological, diagnostic, or therapeutic services. Physicians are paid only for medical services rendered. They are not paid for the so-called "technical component" that is prevalent in the U.S. today. For twenty years, Canada's top-down control worked to keep the health-care-spending-to-GDP ratio well below the rate in the U.S. The tide has turned, though, and Canada is struggling with major cost increases.

The numbers are somewhat skewed because Canada, like some other countries, does not include long-term care institutional costs, many noninstitutional care costs, and prescription drugs in its health care budget. These costs are listed under the social services budget or are paid for by patients. The U.S. most comprehensively folds all health care and long-term care costs into its reporting of health care expenditures.

The strengths of the Canadian system are its universal access and simple single-payer structure, which saves millions in administrative costs compared to the multiple-payer system in the U.S. The Canadian system also effectively controls technological acquisition and physician and hospital fees, and offers universal coverage that does not change substantially or disappear when a person changes jobs. However, the Canadian system also suffers from a growing queuing problem, diminished innovation, and rising costs that may soon rival those in the U.S. Moreover, the single-payer system casts the die for top-down control, which is not compatible with the values of most Americans.

Generally, most polls indicate that Canadians seem satisfied with their system. There are socioeconomic differences between Canada and the U.S., but it appears that much of the public's satisfaction comes from the knowledge that everyone is covered. Each person has a primary-care physician, every individual can obtain emergency care, and no person is bankrupted by catastrophic illness.

ALL FACE AGING PROBLEM

With the virtual elimination of dreaded diseases such as smallpox, polio, measles, and tuberculosis, and advancements in life-prolonging technology, people are living longer. This has placed an increasing demand on every health care system in the world. As a result, governments are scrambling to develop cost-containment strategies. Their methods vary widely because they must be compatible with the political policies and social values of the given country. This is a key point because it is precisely this difference in social and political values that separates and defines the U.S. system as unique in the world. It is also the reason that, while we can borrow some of the components of other nations' health care systems, the values and ideals within the U.S. must ultimately dictate how the system here is reformed.

THE DOUBLE-EDGED SWORD

We Americans like to think of ourselves as the freest people on earth. We like our government, in general, to play as small a part as possible in our daily lives, including health care. This ultimate trust in the individual and competitive marketplace, manifests itself in our lack of centralized national education, transportation, and health care financing and administrative structures. It is this distinction that separates us from most other nations. However, the price we pay for the distinction is higher costs.

Yet, European nations, Canada, New Zealand, Japan, and the other countries utilizing some sort of governmental control, pay a reverse sort of price. While these countries have managed to control costs better than the U.S., their top-down approach causes other problems. In countries where payments to hospitals and physicians have been regulated on a salary or other budget-approved method, efficiency in health care delivery has sometimes dropped and the unwieldy and enervating queuing systems have developed. More important, most countries utilizing top-down control are experiencing a slowing of

the natural evolution of health care compared to the U.S.,
especially in terms of technological and other breakthroughs. The U.S. remains the world leader in the development of high-tech medical equipment, pharmaceuticals
and treatment and diagnostic modalities, and in the creation of new financing and delivery concepts.

As a result, patients from Europe, Canada, and other
countries, who tire of the queuing systems, or who seek
specialized services, pursue care in the U.S. In effect, the
state-of-the-art status of health care that the U.S. has acts
as a "safety valve" for much of the rest of the world. The
catch is that usually only the wealthy can afford to make
the trip to the U.S. for treatment. One sobering thought
is that if the U.S. accepts stringent top-down controls,
which have repressed innovation elsewhere, there may be
no similar backup system for U.S. citizens.

In recent years, states such as California have taken
on another burden—illegal immigrants. Many of these
undocumented people come to the U.S. only to receive
health care. Sophisticated underground networks assist
them in fraudulently obtaining eligibility for services.
Many cross the border to give birth, thereby creating an
obligation on states to care for their U.S.-born children.

RATIONING CARE

While government-controlled systems have managed
to keep a lid on costs, most have done so by rationing
care. For example, pharmaceuticals are not covered under
the Canadian system. In the past decade, Germany,
Denmark, Italy, the Netherlands, Portugal, Greece, and
many other countries systematically removed several drugs

and some services from coverage. In the mid-1980s, the United Kingdom eliminated the right of adults to receive eye glasses and in 1988, the right to free dental checkups and sight tests was also abolished. Dental charges were increased. Similar increases occurred in Germany.

However, since Japanese physicians are allowed to prescribe and dispense pharmaceutical products, which remain high-profit items despite recent governmental reforms, Japan has developed one of the highest per capita consumption of drugs in the world, exceeding that of the U.S. by about 13 percent.

In Germany, per diem hospital reimbursement methods and the fact that German hospitals are prohibited from offering outpatient care, provide the incentives that make the average German patient's hospital stay one of the longest in the world.

This transfer of costs from the public to the private domain has had a two-fold effect. First, it has saved money for the public sector by subtly moving costs to the private sector. Second, as privatization forces people to come face-to-face with the real cost of health care, they have voluntarily reduced their consumption. This fact underscores the belief that any meaningful reform in the U.S. must build on incentives for personal accountability in regard to health care choices.

Another conclusion that can be drawn from examining international health care systems is that administrative costs are less in countries with single-payer or simplified payment systems. Some experts have predicted that if the U.S. adopted a single-collector, single-payer system like Canada's, the resulting savings in administrative costs would be enough to pay for the millions of Americans currently lacking coverage. Yet, in doing so, the U.S. system would undoubtedly lose its competitive edge, its

broad scope of consumer choices and the benefits of pluralism.

The challenge is before us. The ideal reform must
find a way to allow for a simplified financing system while
still maintaining strong incentives for innovation and efficiency. At the same time, we must find a way to control
costs, without creating arbitrary queuing systems or sti-
fling disincentives. Ironically, most of the other countries
mentioned are struggling with the same issues, but from
the opposite end. Nearly all of them are undergoing vary-
ing reforms to rekindle innovation through privatization
and other means.

Yet as those countries move, albeit slowly, toward a
more pluralistic financing structure of public and private
payers, common sense tells us that the U.S. cannot solve
its problems by moving toward a more monolithic system.
Rather than looking for others to lead, the U.S. must
forge ahead and find an innovative solution as it has
historically done in business and social matters.

A NEW PARADIGM

Part of the challenge is to understand our own limits.
No country in the world has higher expectations for its
health care system than the U.S. We are satisfied with
nothing less than the best and latest technology available,
administered by specialists in state-of-the-art facilities. At
the same time, we believe rising health care expenditures
are unacceptable. It is clear that we must find a way to
bring about a better balance between what is demanded,
what is needed, what is ultimately provided, and how it is

paid for. But do not misunderstand—this does not mean that the quality of health care should fall under a cost control axe.

The larger question, of course, is how can the country contain costs without accepting top-down governmental control? The answer cannot be found by mimicking or duplicating a foreign system. Instead, the answer—the health care solution—calls for an entirely new paradigm based on incentives rather than control-oriented directives.

Health care in the U.S. is neither solely private, nor solely public. However, the public influence has been increasing since the passage of Medicare and Medicaid. To disregard powerful market forces in favor of governmental control is to give up when the key to the solution is within reach. The fact is, if competitive market forces are properly channeled through reconfigured and re-aligned incentives, they will act to both contain costs and drive quality and innovation. At the core of the new paradigm must be a system carefully structured to harness the dynamic power of constructive marketplace forces.

INCENTIVES DEFINE SYSTEM

Regardless of the type of health care system, it is the internal incentives that ultimately form the face and define the quality of that system. Uniformly, in countries where government limits provider payments and rations resources, providers lack the competitive incentives to provide state-of-the-art service and the quality of health care is defined in different terms.

But, providing proper incentives for providers won't be enough. To be successful, the new model must also include congruent incentives for third-party payers and the public. In order to reach the goal of universal access, third-party payers must be given the incentive to cover all people, not just those who are low-risk. At the same time, incentives must be put into place that require consumers to accept responsibility for their health care decisions so resources aren't wasted, high-cost specialists and technology aren't needlessly utilized and life-style choices are made judiciously with health in mind.

PERSONAL ACCOUNTABILITY

To support this system, it is vital that other U.S. policies encourage the philosophy of health promotion. For example, consumers of tobacco and other products detrimental to human health cannot be subsidized by the government. They must be treated much like gas-guzzling cars, which have been recognized as wasteful and subjected to special "luxury" taxes at the time of purchase.

Much more effort must be put into educating the public about the direct correlation between life-styles and health costs. The numbers are sobering. In 1992, nearly $171 billion, accounting for nearly one out of every four dollars spent on health care in the U.S., went to treating victims of drug abuse, violence and other medical conditions that could have been avoided, according to the American Medical Association. Other factors included the failure to use such life-saving technology as seat belts and smoke detectors, failure to get routine medical checkups that could detect cancer and other treatable diseases, and having unprotected sex.

**Leading preventable causes of death
representing 63% of all deaths**

United States: 1980

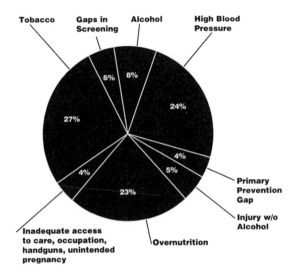

SOURCE: Robert Amler and H. Bruce Dull, *Closing the Gap: The Burden of Unnecessary Illness*, Oxford University Press, New York, 1987.

The cost to every person in the nation for these irresponsible actions is substantial. It is imperative that a system of personal accountability be established so that each person fully realizes his or her responsibility to adapt a healthier life-style.

CHARTING A NEW COURSE

The next seven chapters provide a blueprint for the new system, based on properly aligned incentives that seize the advantages offered by competitive market collaboration.

While acknowledging the strengths and weaknesses of health care systems around the world, we must chart our own course toward a new solution.

FINANCING
THE SYSTEM

▼

Any meaningful reform of the health care system must begin with the way it is financed. Financing is not only the foundation of any health care system, it plays a major role in defining it. Once the financing mechanism is in place and the payment methodologies are established, the delivery elements follow. The policy and practical procedures established during the financing stage will set the

stage for reimbursing plans and providers. Distribution of
funds to providers will dictate the way services are organized and delivered.

At first glance, the financing choice is intriguing
because of the possibilities. In reality, however, financing
options for the U.S. system are limited by our unique sociological and political expectations and demands. For example, a strict top-down system, funded entirely by the
government, which in turn restricts services and payments
to providers, has slim chance for acceptance here. To date,
the U.S. has been unwilling to make the trade-off—that
is, the loss of individual choice and diminishment of
provider innovation and initiative for restricted access,
utilization controls, and lower costs.

THE INVISIBLE COST

Paying for health care services began as an individual
choice. People either paid for services they needed, or
chose to forego them. A self-imposed rationing system
was generated, based on the price of the service provided.
Thus, the financing of health care began in a way no
different than the financing of any private industry.

In the 1940s, insurance companies and other third-
party carriers changed the financing and payment mentality forever. Rather than paying the direct costs of health
care services, individuals began paying periodic premiums, and thus isolated themselves from the real costs of
financing their health care.

Employer-paid insurance, Medicare, and Medicaid
radically altered the direct financing of health care since
World War II. The self-imposed rationing system was
obliterated. These new financing mechanisms were based

on the cost of the services rendered, regardless of what that cost happened to be. The full consequences of this change in financing were not felt immediately, because technology was still at a rudimentary stage of development and alternatives for treating patients were severely limited. Therefore, the cost of governmental programs and employer-paid insurance were relatively modest. For a time, it continued to reflect the true cost of the system. As services, facilities and technology began to expand in the 1970s and 1980s, health care costs raced into high gear.

Population with health care coverage*

United States: 1984-1990 (000,000)

Year	Total Population	Public & Private Health Care Coverage		Private Health Care Coverage	
		Total Persons	% of Population	Total Persons	% of Population
1984	233.5	202.1	86.6%	177.4	76.0%
1985	235.5	204.2	86.7	180.1	76.5
1986	238.2	204.4	85.8	180.1	75.6
1987	240.4	208.2	86.6	183.2	76.2
1988	243.1	211.6	87.1	188.4	77.5
1989	244.9	213.6	87.2	189.0	77.2
1990	248.9	214.0	86.1	182.2	73.2

* Totals may not add due to duplicate counting and rounding.

SOURCE: Health Insurance Association of America, *Source Book of Health Insurance Data, 1991*, Washington, D.C..

A GROWING FAULT LINE

The federal government reacted to rising health care costs by cutting back on payments to providers and shifting costs to state and local governments. Third-party financiers moved to cut costs by decreasing provider payments on one end and squeezing out so-called "high-risk" groups of consumers on the other. However, employers made no similar retrenchment in the services provided their workers, or curbs on the expanding size of the employee benefit packages they offered.

As financing assumed a "less-and-less" mentality, benefits and coverage took on a "more-and-more" rationale. The result has been a widening chasm between expectation and reality—a rapidly widening fault line of divergent philosophies that today threatens to topple the entire system.

It is impossible to finance a system when the demands and indicators are all moving in different directions. The challenge that lies ahead is to develop a financing mechanism that will align our expectations of health care with the reality of its costs, while at the same time remaining harmonious with accepted social values.

INDIVIDUAL INVOLVEMENT

Any successful financing mechanism must call into play individual responsibility and involvement regarding health status and health care decisions. Privately funded health care, through employers and third-party carriers, is logical and consistent with past philosophies. Employers have accepted a major responsibility for health care coverage since the 1960s. Future financing should be based on a continuation and expansion of that existing mechanism to maintain pluralistic financing. It would be difficult politically to transfer all health care costs to the government because of the significant tax rate hike that would be required.

For nearly thirty years, however, government has accepted responsibility for the aged and some of the economically disadvantaged who are not covered by employers. This pluralistic approach offers the best promise for achieving the two primary goals of the new paradigm—universal access and affordable cost.

100% EMPLOYER-SPONSORED COVERAGE

One of the most serious problems facing the present system is the increasing inability of middle-class workers to afford health care. In 1992, the majority of those losing health care coverage in the U.S. were working people of middle incomes—often employed by small companies or self-employed—who could no longer afford the high cost of coverage. Such a distressing trend must be halted.

The most effective way to guarantee access to health care for all employees is through universal employer coverage of a uniform benefit package. This is hardly a new idea—that all employers be required to furnish coverage for their employees—but it has recently gained approval from major employer organizations. Organizations such as The American Chamber of Commerce, for example, have recently become more receptive to the idea of nationwide employer-sponsored coverage. With this type of coverage, portability barriers are removed and loss of coverage, job-lock, and preexisting conditions would no longer be problems.

TAX INCENTIVES FOR SMALL EMPLOYERS

The vast majority of large employers nationwide already provide employee coverage within their benefit packages, so in these cases there would be little change. However, there is a well-founded concern that a mandate would create undue hardship for small and low-wage employers, perhaps even driving them out of business. This concern can be met by providing tax incentives, tax credits or direct subsidies for qualifying small and new businesses. The federal income tax system is a ready-made vehicle to implement such a program. For example, if a company's taxable income falls below a certain amount on a graduated scale established by Congress, it would qualify for tax breaks. For every dollar the company pays in health care, the government could match it dollar for dollar. A similar scale could be established for self-employed workers. The scale itself should be established through the political process, with the interests of small-business owners and selfemployed workers given primary weight.

Another approach would be to limit the amount small and low-wage employers pay for health insurance. Subsidies to cover the shortfall could be made up from general tax revenues or from other employers.

It is logical that the concept of employer-sponsored coverage be accepted because it is the best and most readily available option we have to ensure universal coverage for all employees and their uninsured dependents.

THE UNEMPLOYED

To provide seamless health care for everyone, the system must also account for the unemployed. For those workers who have been laid off or terminated, employers could be required to continue coverage for an established length of time, perhaps 180 days. Before that time has expired, the government would decide whether the individual meets the eligibility standards for Medicare or Medicaid. Those able to pay for continued coverage could be required to do so.

For those employees who voluntarily quit their jobs, the provisions set forth under the Omnibus Budget Reconciliation Act of 1986 could apply. They would have the option to buy coverage from their immediate former employer, but they would have to pay the full premium, plus two percent. In other words, these people would be guaranteed coverage if they could afford it, or they would be covered through the governmental program if they couldn't pay the premiums.

INSURANCE REFORM AND UNIVERSAL ACCESS

Employer-sponsored coverage will achieve universal access in the private sector by eliminating destructive, exclusionary insurance practices. Squeezed by rising health costs on one hand and increased consumer expectations on the other, third-party carriers have reacted by creating predatory practices to enhance their positions. Often, these practices claim higher priority than serving the public interest or the long-term financial viability of the health care system. As mentioned before, these practices include extraordinary-experience rating, denying coverage to individuals or small groups for a variety of reasons—such as pre-existing conditions, place and type of employment, age, sex preference—and red-lining (arbitrarily locking out) individuals and groups.

The purpose of the non-issuance and nonrenewal of policies, exorbitant premiums, and refusal to cover certain groups is to eliminate these "high-risk" people from the insurance market. This effort to drive "undesirables" from coverage has worked well for carriers. Each year thousands of working Americans lose their health care insurance.

Insurance was created to spread the risk and utilize the benefits gained from the probabilities of large numbers. Community rating was the original foundation for insurance. Exclusionary and predatory practices are inconsistent with this concept. If allowed to continue, these self-interest practices will threaten the viability of private insurance in the eyes of the public. Without a realignment of market incentives, they will continue to multiply in a variety of increasingly clever forms. Ultimately, they will undermine the entire third-party payer system and create the opportunity for government to take over the financing and payment functions.

Universal employer-sponsored coverage of a uniform benefit package eliminates the conflict by realigning market incentives and by producing a predictable, risk-spreading financial resource. Reforms including guaranteed policy issue and renewal, the abolishment of pre-existing condition exclusions, and the return to community rating are vital. The economic pressures that have caused the exclusionary mutations will be replaced by equitable competition. Health insurance then can revert to community rating, engendering equity, increased access, and affordability. Quality, service and price will be comparable for the public.

BALANCING CHOICE AND COST

Pluralism—joint financing by government and the private sector—is already an accepted tenant of the financing system. Although it implies individual decision making, it does not mean unbridled choice. There is a misconception in the U.S. that the health care system should offer unrestricted and opened-ended choice. We have historically placed a high value on certain choices, especially the freedom to chose hospitals and physicians. The rapid growth and popularity of health maintenance organizations and other capitated systems, however, suggests that unlimited choice of doctors may not be as important as previously believed.

What must be understood, is that for every choice, there is a corresponding cost. There is ample evidence to show that while choice is important, at some point it becomes secondary to cost considerations. At that point, people willingly accept a restricted number of choices, provided that access and quality remain acceptable.

Some individuals, of course, will have more options than others due to their economic status. Wealthy people may choose to enhance their choices by paying more, a reality that has always been an accepted part of the free-enterprise system and the American way. But clearly, the system should not subsidize this increased utilization, as it currently does through the taxing system. With the plan, an individual who decides to go outside of the system he or she is enrolled in would not be allowed to deduct the additional costs from his or her taxes. This concept could be extended to apply to premiums paid for benefits exceeding the uniform benefit package.

Consider, for example, John's case, which is all too common today. John is a 69-year-old retiree who was a vice president at a national real estate firm's regional office. John had been an executive most of his professional life and was financially well prepared for retirement. Because he had saved conscientiously over the years, he and his wife were able to live a comfortable life on approximately $250,000 a year.

John, no longer on the company's health insurance plan, continued to receive medical care from his primary physician, a cardiologist. Because he had rarely seen other doctors in the last few years, he felt comfortable with this physician and saw him for everything from cardiac problems to the occasional case of strep throat—all at the same fee of $75 per office visit. John was over 65 years of age, so Medicare—funded by taxes—paid for his visits regardless of the nature of his ailment and in spite of the cost.

The misuse of Medicaid funds occurs in a somewhat similar way. Those who use Medicaid—the poor—often receive health services many consider to be more extensive than is necessary. The case of Mary, a 39-year-old, is a prime example.

Mary contracted a bone disease after stepping on a nail. Her treatment consisted of six weeks of antibiotics given intravenously. After being seen in the emergency room, Mary remained in the hospital so that the I.V. drugs could be initiated. Once the I.V. was started, Mary could have returned home for the rest of the treatment's course. If this had occurred, a home nurse would have been dispatched to make a brief house call each day—a service that costs less than $50 per visit. However, since Medicaid does not pay for home health care, Mary had to stay in the hospital for the entire six weeks at a cost of approximately $350 a day (just to use the room). By standardizing care, the plan would ensure that impractical, unneeded care— as was provided in Mary's case—would no longer occur.

PROMOTION OF WELLNESS

Much of this problem stems from our lack of emphasis on preventative health care practices, such as the promotion of wellness. The financing and payment system has come to be based on the consumption of services and resources. Programs designed to reduce consumption, such as healthy diets and exercise, are more often treated as fads that do not produce immediate savings. As a consequence, the financiers of such services dropped the programs or converted them to cafeteria-type benefit plans, which employees value more highly because they have a choice of benefits.

This is a mind-set and condition that must be reversed. The old truism that "an ounce of prevention is worth a pound of cure" is applicable here. Preventative practices must be re-established as a top priority among the public and health care providers, both for health and cost reasons.

The "do-more" incentives that drive providers toward increasing specialized services—many of them unnecessary—must be reversed. The goals of providers must be realigned to coincide with those of their patients', namely a mutual focus and emphasis on prevention, timely intervention and wellness. Employee-sponsored coverage, coupled with redesigned provider networks described in the chapter on the delivery system, will achieve this end.

NO DUPLICITOUS MESSAGES

The federal government has been the major culprit in sending mixed signals about preventative health practices. While several examples come to mind, the most glaring is the consumption of tobacco products. As previously mentioned, it is inconsistent for the government to issue warnings about the dangers of tobacco and simultaneously subsidize the producers of tobacco products. Government cannot continue to convey duplicitous messages. If individuals wish to consume products known to be detrimental to their health and others', they should pay for that privilege. They should not be protected from the ensuing consequences or responsibility. The best way to approach this problem is by instituting a user's fee at the point of purchase. Similarly, taxes on alcohol, hand guns, and other potentially harmful consumer products should be paid at the time of purchase.

A recent Wall Street Journal/NBC poll found overwhelming support for increased taxes on cigarettes, alcohol, and other products considered health hazards. Of those surveyed, 70 percent said they could accept at least a $2 tax increase on a pack of cigarettes and 87 percent said they could accept a $1 tax increase on a quart of liquor or wine.

The funds collected through these "user fees" should be channeled to help support the provision of health care for the uninsured. It is time that those who create such huge costs to the health care system accept their individual responsibility to help pay the price.

SEAMLESS HEALTH CARE

While the private/public financing partnership ensures coverage for employees and their dependents and those enrolled in Medicare and Medicaid programs, there will inevitably be individuals still without coverage. No nation in the world is able to provide front-end enrollment and coverage for every resident. People who fall through the cracks include the homeless and transitory, mentally ill, and others who, for whatever reason, choose not to be a part of the system. California, Florida, Texas, and New York have many illegal immigrants in this category.

To provide seamless health care—a primary goal of the new paradigm—we must establish a system of providing a health care safety net for this population. The financing of health care for these people is difficult to determine on a pre-paid capitation basis. Since the number of individuals who fall into this category is relatively small, the best way to provide coverage is to finance their care on a fee-for-service basis for the providers who treat them or to establish payment arrangements with safety net providers who render a high proportion of the services. Financing should come from general revenues and be included in society's overall obligation to provide health care for all residents. Payments for care rendered to illegal immigrants should be a federal government responsibility since immigration is administered at the national level under federal laws.

It must be recognized that these individuals may not participate in the preventative promotion of wellness and other services that will be given to enrolled persons. However, it would be prudent to provide education on preventative health care measures to these individuals at their point of entry. A financial incentive may also be worthy of consideration. They should be given the opportunity to enroll in an appropriate program so they can benefit from the full scale of services available.

The bottom line is that to achieve seamless health care, the financing for disadvantaged people in this category cannot be ignored. The cost must be factored into the system in advance, as part of the overall financing program.

Primary financing of health care by each individual is unrealistic. So is a single-payer system whereby government picks up the entire tab; the adage, "If it ain't broke, don't fix it," applies here. The present private/public financing partnership, with the added dimension of employer-mandated coverage for employees, offers the best solution for financing the new system.

THE PAYMENT SYSTEM

▼

Once the new financing system is established, a method of paying providers must follow. The payment system is also essential to the success of the new paradigm. While the pluralistic financing system outlined in the last chapter ensures universal access, the payment system and delivery network must tackle the overriding problem of escalating costs.

Specifically, the challenge is to design a new payment system that re-aligns the existing perverse incentives, which have left consumers, carriers, and providers, with differing and often opposing goals. This critical step has been left unaddressed by most proposed reforms because it calls for difficult choices and a modification in carrier and provider roles. Making these choices requires the political and social will that is emerging as we recognize that without major change, the system is inevitably headed toward meltdown and governmental control.

ECONOMIC PREDICTABILITY

The first requirement of the new payment system is that payments must be made to integrated provider networks in a predictable and programmed manner. Without this element, the system will not escape the most damaging of the incentives—the motivation of providers to do more to make more. The new system must eradicate the incentives that leave providers constantly searching for ways to carve out new territories, unbundle existing services into multiple, individually priced services, and refer and recommend an ever-increasing number of services to consumers for a charge. The new plan must include fixed payments for provider groups, which then take on responsibility and accountability for the health care of specific persons and for their own economic survival.

This concept virtually reverses the present system. Currently, we pay for fragmentation, with little accountability from those who receive payments to collectively become more efficient. Increasingly, providers and carriers are recognizing the short-sightedness of this scheme, and the long-term devastation it causes. This situation must be replaced with a new method of payment that provides economic discipline and predictability, based on the availability of a finite amount of money.

The new payment system must be designed so that it creates compatible incentives for consumers, carriers, and providers. These must also be harmonious with the incentives and philosophies of the financing and delivery systems, as well as society as a whole.

TWO APPROACHES TO PAYMENT

Assuming a fixed annual payment is made to community health networks (the network concept is explained in the next chapter), there are two ways of approaching payment in a pluralistic system. The first is a modified fee-for-service method. The second is a negotiated payment to providers to cover all services included in the uniform benefit package. Called "full capitation," this concept provides for a periodic per capita payment on an annual basis. This aggregate payment covers an individual for all services included in a uniform benefit package, which defines what care must be provided by the networks each year.

Under the modified fee-for-service scenario, providers render individual or bundled services for set fees. The mechanics of this system include third-party payers making arrangements with individual providers or groups of providers for certain services at a negotiated price. These primary-care provider groups are backed up by other groups comprised of specialists, pharmacists, hospitals, and other providers. Payment contracts are negotiated with the nonprimary-care providers.

The benefit of the fee-for-service option is that the primary provider groups act as the entry point into the entire system. Therefore, they are motivated to minimize the use of the most costly services. This is commonly called a gatekeeper arrangement. The major disadvantage of this system is that providers may have conflicting incentives. The incentive to increasingly provide more services remains for certain providers, such as specialists, hospitals and many other providers. Further, the primary-care groups, which are the entry point for the entire system, may not have incentives that are compatible with providing total health care services for the entire population. Primary-care practitioners may transfer "costly" or "undesirable" patients, encourage certain patients to enroll in other plans, transfer services to other providers, or make inappropriate referrals which serve their financial interests. In such cases, the shifting of responsibility may occur because the entire provider network is not integrated. All these types of distortions can occur, if the primary gatekeeper and other providers in the chain are not compatibly motivated.

How does Canada handle the challenge? Canada essentially has loosely organized independent practice associations of physicians and franchised hospitals. It does not effectively control either the consumption of resources, or the utilization of non-hospital services, except by limiting the availability of institutional facilities and technology. Canadian physicians, for the most part, are paid on a fee-for-service basis, even though some doctors are paid a salary. Consequently, incompatible and often opposing incentives persist within the system and some providers still strive to continually expand their service bases. This fact, coupled with the absence of local integration of providers, has kept Canada from achieving desired cost containment goals in recent years.

THE FULL-CAPITATION METHOD

The second option of payment, the "full-capitation" method, is the better long-term choice for the United States. This system minimizes the reliance on fee-for-service arrangements. Instead, community health networks of providers are paid a set amount per individual, which covers that patient for all services defined in the uniform benefit package.

The results of this change would be enormous. First and foremost, it would eliminate the providers' incentive to engage in techno-turf wars and the mad scramble to provide more and more services. In a fully capitated system, with a finite amount of money flowing into the provider network, conserving resources and providing services efficiently and economically, will be the incentives. In effect, a bottom-up global budget will result.

HOW CAPITATION AFFECTS PROVIDERS

A fully capitated system will affect providers' attitudes and behavior in a number of ways. First, it eliminates the isolation and false sense of security that now envelops the industry. It is a common belief among most providers that they efficiently deliver services and individually are not the cause of rising costs and growing health care inaccessibility. Ironically, most hospitals are improving efficiency,

providing more tests, units of service and therapies per
employee than ever before. However, more and more is
being done.

Under a fully capitated system of integrated networks, providers must answer directly to their network
and to the consumers, prompting a re-allocation of resources and services. Community health networks will determine the amount and location of facilities, technology,
and personnel. Independent, self-generating payments
will no longer be made for such things as too many MRIs,
lab tests, and diagnostic workups. The number of surgeries will be replaced with less invasive and more conserv-
ative options when the surgeries do not generate more
revenue.

Under such an arrangement, the providers will be
motivated to give educational, preventative services as
well as other support services that will result in healthier
clients, less demand for provider services, and less strain
on the limited financial funds available. Members of a
community health network will need to manage their
costs so that the total capitation payments are adequate.
Also, patients' sensitivity to cost can be augmented by the
use of deductibles and co-payments at the time they receive services.

The duplication of high-tech services, specialized
services, and diagnostic technology will be eliminated
because there will be no financial incentive for their
existence. Consolidation of resources such as cardiovascular services will produce concentrated volumes,
resulting in lower costs and higher quality. Community
health networks will survive only if they respond to what
clients want. Since people will choose annually whether
they wish to remain with a community health network,

the shoe is put on the other foot. Consumers become the dominant force in the selection process. Community health networks will be entities of collaboration that must appeal to consumers on the basis of quality, service and price. Universal access to a uniform benefit package allow consumers to choose the community health network of preference.

HOW CAPITATION AFFECTS CARRIERS

This system will have a similar effect on third-party payors. Since community health networks will get a single payment that covers all services, there will be no need for such costly administrative duties as hospital bill auditing and outside utilization reviews.

With the current system, even the treatments recommended for patients by providers are evaluated by the middle layer of insurance carriers and auditors, who decide which services will be covered. In these cases, the provider must often telephone the payer and obtain reimbursement authorization from its personnel, some of which are neither nurses nor physicians. Other insurance carriers screen patients and determine which provider, if any, to whom the patient should be assigned. It is also common for a health care professional, hired by the payer, to continually review the services a doctor provides throughout the patient's course of treatment. Another review of the patient's record may take place after treatment ends, to determine whether appropriate care was provided in a timely manner. Additional functions of the middle layer include securing second opinions and other monitoring procedures.

Usually, when the payer receives a final bill which exceeds a pre-determined amount, auditors review it, yet again, to be sure the charges are in line with the services that were provided. Medicare and Medicaid representatives also perform additional on-site audits designed to check the intermediaries (companies that administer governmental programs). Whether the payer is an insurance company or the government, this system is clearly a costly one in terms of monetary and human resources. These excessive measures gobble up more than $1.25 billion annually!

This massive waste of public and private dollars will be reduced significantly under the new system. If the community health networks do not deliver what they promise, their enrolled clients will simply switch networks during an annual enrollment period. Therefore, there will be no value added by a middle layer of checking, monitoring, and auditing the system. Rather than being wasted in meaningless bureaucratic pursuits, this money can go into the provision of preventative, diagnostic, and therapeutic services. Internal economic discipline will replace external control agents.

To achieve universal access, a fully capitated system must also encompass new standards for carriers and the carrier function within consolidated community health networks. These must include the reforms mentioned earlier. These negative practices would be eliminated through a universal-access requirement. No carrier or community health network would be permitted to exclude any individual who wishes to enroll and receive the coverage contained in the uniform benefit package.

More than 1,300 carriers and insurance companies were in operation in the U.S. in 1992. That number would drop under the new system because those profiting solely from their highly perfected, cherry-picking practices would not meet the underwriting criteria. Fewer carriers would result in less duplication of costly middle-layer bureaucracies, claims processing, and the other procedural costs that occur in the market today. Fewer agents would also depend on health coverage commissions for a portion of their income.

The biggest advantage to the surviving carriers is that their role and importance within the health care equation changes. They become major players in the negotiations with employers and providers. Their role will include negotiations emphasizing accountability, the deployment of resources, total costs, and outcomes. These things do not occur today because each company is trying to look out for itself. They have little regard for what happens on the delivery side (except to ratchet down payments) as long as they can obtain money from the financing side to cover their expenses, profits, and discounted payments to providers.

The new payment system eliminates the incentives that cause third-party carriers to scale down payments to providers and hammer them into submission through external controls. Carriers will no longer be able to squeeze out "undesirable" patients in their scramble for higher profits within a shifting market. Carriers will instead become motivated to put the patients' interests first.

It is likely that most carriers and community health networks will consolidate to form a comprehensive organization that handles all functions for consumers. This concentration will increase productivity, make choices easier for consumers, and give them greater influence over their health support system.

HOW CAPITATION RATE IS NEGOTIATED

The capitation rate will be negotiated annually on a group basis, with large employers negotiating on behalf of themselves and small employers and individuals banding together in health alliances to purchase coverage collectively. The negotiations with carriers and community health networks, or both, will reach a level that is acceptable to all parties if the proper elements are in place. Guaranteed access to a uniform benefit package for every person provides for a precise bottom-up budget and, therefore, economic predictability. A well-defined uniform benefit package guarantees that consumers, providers, and payers know exactly what to expect in terms of services and resources.

In the event that an employer or alliance cannot reach agreement on a capitation rate with a community health network, it would have the option of paying the community health network the weighted average price of competing community health networks. Persons covered by the employer or alliance would pay the difference if they chose the higher priced community health network.

The concept of managed collaboration is pivotal here, and will infuse the system with the dynamics of a competitive marketplace where it does not now exist. Community health networks will be forced to compete against each other—in the classic American style of competition in an open market—on matters of quality, service and price. This will prevent the fragmentation of services, cost shifting, inconsistencies among benefits, and manipulative practices.

OPEN ENROLLMENT PERIOD

An annual open-enrollment period is essential because it greatly enhances the competitive dynamics of the system. If an employee or individual becomes unhappy with the service or price of a given community health network, he or she can switch networks the following year. This puts pressure on all providers within a community health network to perform at peak efficiency, both economically and professionally.

For capitation to work, we have to be willing to accept the reality that networks do not have an inherent constitutional right to survive; they have an opportunity to succeed or to fail. Similarly, each resident's right to health care does not guarantee unlimited choice—it ensures reasonable choice.

Unless we allow for the opportunity for failure, competition will be unsuccessful. Will the failure of one community health network destroy health care? No. In urban areas, where a number of networks will compete, it is unlikely that a failing network will collapse overnight. Most will falter gradually. But if one folds suddenly, other community health networks in the area will compete for the business at their published or newly negotiated rates.

WORKERS' COMPENSATION

A further obstacle to implementing the new order is the fact that payment for most health services is inextricably tied to the source that mandates the need for the service. If that sounds confusing and bureaucratic, it's because it is just that. All the same, it is an important concept to understand because it is the source of a serious problem. Here's how it works.

If you are injured while on the job, payment for your health care probably comes from workers' compensation. However, if you are injured in an automobile or at home, your respective auto or home insurance covers you. If you just plain get sick, your health insurance covers you. If you think about it logically for a moment, the entire system appears absurd. Billions of dollars are expended annually by insurance companies, lawyers, and others just to determine which entity should pay the bill!

The point is, if health is to become a right and everyone is to have equitable access to a uniform benefit package, it is vital that all health services be consolidated into a single health policy. Under the new paradigm, it will not matter whether you were injured or became sick at work, in your car, or at home. One policy will cover all contingencies. Not only does this eliminate duplication of costly systems, regulations, audits and reviews, but in many instances health care would be removed from the tort system. This would have the tremendously positive effect of greatly reducing litigation involving automobile and home owner's insurance, and especially workers' compensation.

Today, small employers are paying up to 15 percent of their payroll to cover workers' compensation programs. In most cases, more than 20 percent of their workers' compensation premiums are for health benefits and related expenses.

By consolidating workers' compensation health benefits into round-the-clock employer-paid health insurance, employers will reduce their costs considerably and provide their employees with better benefits at the same time. This consolidation will produce a win-win arrangement

**Workers' compensation medical treatment costs –
15.9% of every premium dollar is for medical treatment**

California – 1992

Medical Treatment by Provider

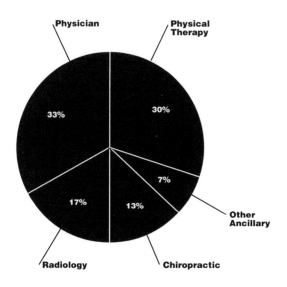

SOURCE: California Workers' Compensation Institute, State Compensation Insurance Fund and California Medical Association, 1992.

for everyone, except for those who have made a lucrative business out of workers' compensation. The money now being drained off for the administrative and legal costs could be used to promote good health practices and provide increased health services.

A round-the-clock policy is the answer to solving the access and uniform benefit failures that now exist. If people can receive necessary health care regardless of the cause (work, accident, etc.), they can use their regular health plan. In addition, providers could avoid the stress of litigation and navigating a notoriously inefficient bureaucratic system, maintain continuity of care, and promote cost effectiveness.

A tremendous benefit of the new model, made possible through capitation payments, is that workers' compensation costs would be reduced because all injuries and sicknesses, irrespective of whether they are work-related, would be covered under the uniform benefit package. The substantial tort expenses and administrative nightmares associated with workers' compensation health benefits would also be reduced to a minimum.

To a lesser degree, savings could be generated if the health benefits paid to providers as the result of auto accidents were included in the uniform benefit package.

Workers' compensation costs
California – 1992

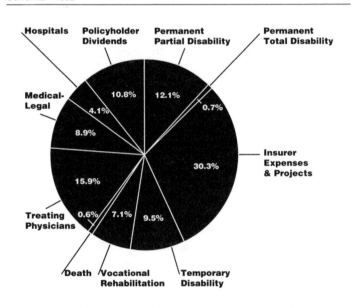

SOURCE: California Economic Summit, California State Legislature, Sacramento, 1993.

HELP FOR SMALL EMPLOYERS

The new system does not radically alter the requirements of large employers, since most already offer universal employee coverage. However, provisions to help small and new employers and the self-employed must be addressed because they will experience a net increase in costs. To balance this new business cost, government must provide a tax credit, subsidy or similar off-set, to qualifying low-wage employers. This should include a fixed, phase-in program for new low-wage businesses to give them time to provide the services and benefits and allow them to survive economically during their start-up period.

Average employer contribution to workers' health plans by firm size

United States: 1992

Firm Size	Workers w/Group Health at Least Partially Paid by Employer (000)	Average Employer Contribution
Fewer than 10 employees	4.8	$2,093
10-24 employees	4.3	2,002
25-99 employees	7.9	2,027
100-499 employees	10.7	2,029
500-999 employees	4.6	2,115
1,000 or more employees	32.1	2,213

SOURCE: Employee Benefit Research Institute, *Special Report*, "Sources of Health Insurance and Characteristics of the Uninsured," Issue Brief Number 133, January 1993, Washington, D.C.

Today, the cost of health care is proportionately highest for low wage and small businesses. Under the new system, the elimination of predatory carrier practices, regressive payment practices, administrative overhead, and legal wastes, coupled with tax incentives, will cause employee health costs for these groups to drop dramatically.

THE DELIVERY SYSTEM

The health care delivery system in the U.S. operates like a huge consumption machine and, as such, it works well. Driven by the do-more-to-get-more attitude, it has developed a voracious appetite for cash. Providers motivated by misguided governmental policies, compete in a head-long race to deliver more services and technology, instead of concentrating on the production of high-quality, low-cost services and products.

The final, major step toward reforming the health care system will entail a restructuring of the delivery mechanism. A new system, based on a common vision and congruent incentives for all stakeholders, is needed. A system that relies on access through vertically integrated, risk-bearing delivery networks is the most tested and proven solution.

The integrated network concept has gained a groundswell of support in recent years, emerging under a variety of names, including: health maintenance organizations, managed competition, community-care networks, organized delivery systems, and accountable health plans. Although some of these designs have differences, the basic idea is the same. As competing, vertically and horizontally integrated regional networks, they consist of physicians, hospitals, and other providers, who render for pre-determined payments the baseline services required under a defined uniform benefit package.

Community health networks will likely be formed around existing providers and carriers. For example, within a metropolitan area the size of Sacramento, California (approximate population of 1.5 million), it is easy to envision three or four networks, each competing with one another to enroll clients.

While integrated networks will work well in urbanized areas, rural communities generally will not be as easily adaptable to such concepts because of the sparse population, range of providers and limited choices. Simply stated, rural areas must be treated differently from urban centers.

THE INSATIABLE APPETITE

Through the 1980s, the delivery system was dramatically reshaped by providers. Pressures on providers to survive caused a horizontal expansion of the delivery system. Many practitioners purchased equipment and technology, adding technological components to their practices that have become a vital part of their service and financial base. In other instances, small groups of providers created circular arrangements for referrals and the delivery of blocks of services. Some of these led to an abuse of referrals and services.

This proliferation of services, and the concept advanced by providers that these high-tech components are essential to good health, followed the Medicare-generated philosophy that more is better in the consumption of health resources. An insatiable appetite was created on both sides and the delivery system has become a self-generating servant, scurrying to meet expanding, public demands.

TRAGEDY OF THE COMMONS

Three major forces combined in recent years to resist meaningful reform. First, the tragedy of the commons was at work. Although individual providers were basically aware that the payment and delivery system was aiding and abetting the overutilization of resources, most providers had already fought their turf battles and were reluctant to give up hard-won individual positions for the common good.

Instead, providers, feeling besieged by poorly
designed government and insurance efforts to curb costs,
started to "game" the system, and their vision narrowed to
the confines of their individual economic survival. Forced
into a bunker mentality, they strived to work around governmental and insurance regulations and payment cut-
backs to increase services and negotiate payments at the
highest level possible.

Second, while the gap between the haves and have-
nots continued to grow, there was little political motivation to solve the problem. More than 85 percent of voters
were generally satisfied with their health coverage—private or public—and were reluctant to embrace changes.
The elderly stood strongly for Medicare and the insured
voters under sixty-five were unwilling to forfeit their
choices, most of which were through employer-paid coverage. Since the economically disadvantaged and uninsured people lacked significant voting clout, elected
officials were hesitant to tackle reforms. As long as other
public policy issues were more pressing, health care
reform was swept under the rug.

Finally, short-sighted governmental regulations continually missed the mark, focusing primarily on more
standards, increased reporting requirements, and reduced
payments. Rather than change the internal incentives that
were driving providers toward unbundling services and
horizontal expansion, these futile attempts to secure artificial lids on costs backfired.

THE INTEGRATED NETWORK EVOLUTION

The first steps toward collaborative networks were taken
to battle costs more than fifty years ago, led by the Kaiser
Permanente Health Plan in California. Capitation became

a reality and began to influence the way services were delivered. However, it wasn't until the 1970s, when health care costs began to escalate rapidly, that other health maintenance organizations (HMOs), or prepaid capitated plans, began to proliferate. Governmental injections also helped stimulate some HMOs. As the plans grew more established, they were modified in many different ways in response to patient demands. Since 1977, HMO enrollment has grown from covering 3 percent to 15 percent of the population. The number of HMOs has tripled during that time period. It is estimated that more than one-third of the privately insured national population will obtain their care from HMO providers in 1994. By 1995, HMOs will be offered as an option to an estimated 90 percent of all employers nationwide.

Reforms, which are occurring in many parts of the nation, are summarized in the chart showing trends.

However, the change to capitated community health networks is far from universal. Competition among the capitated programs, discounted managed-care programs, and traditional delivery systems is in full swing but economic predictability has a long way to go.

Fearing the potential of capitated networks, opponents fueled the belief that the limited provider networks fail to provide choices and offer inferior service or quality. Although no empirical data exist to show that the quality of care within integrated and capitated networks is inferior to independent care, the myth survived. To this day, it continues to divide providers and patients. Unfortunately, this fiction may represent a psychological obstacle to reforming the system through capitated, integrated networks.

The proof is in the public's actions. If capitated networks were of poor quality or service, no one would enroll. The opposite, however, is true. In California, more

Trends – Health Care in the 21st Century

Components/Issues	Current	Future
Population	Growing cultural diversity	Majority non-white in states and local areas
	Emerging population changes	Aging population with growing influence and intergenerational gap
Economy	Mixture of national and worldwide markets	Worldwide driven markets, decline in U.S. influence, and emphasis on quality
	Majority middle class	Widening of gap between poor and wealthy with disproportionate growth of non-wealthy residents
Information	Differential levels and isolation of information and data	Universal access to integrated information and data
		Public awareness and broad distribution of performance and outcomes data
Technology	Explosion of new technology resulting in expanding consumption of resources	Continued growth in new technology with emphasis on reducing costs and consumption, greater convenience and alternatives
Heath Status	Widening gap between the healthy and the non-healthy	More threats to health status due to behavioral and environmental influences
		New pathology
		New definition of health status and goals
Health Policy and Reform	Inconsistent incrementalism	Equitable access with economic predictability
	Individualized protections and segmentation	Organized health delivery systems which integrate health status, prevention services and cost effectiveness
	Episodic care and intervention	Improving health status, good practices, preventive health and seamless services

(Table continues on following page.)

than 10 million of 32 million residents, are enrolled in a capitated plan with restricted choices and financial penalties for going outside the system. Further, the vast majori-

Trends – Health Care in the 21st Century
(Continued from previous page.)

Components/Issues	Current	Future
Hospitals	Competition and separate interests	Collaboration and partnership; resizing
	Institutional and horizontal focus	Community and vertically integrated focus; coordinated programs to improve health status and deliver services efficiently
		Alternative, non-inpatient emphasis
Hospitals/ Physicians	Independent tracks	Linkages among hospitals and physician groups; shared risks
Labor	Competing units and professions; jurisdictional disputes	Integrated use of resources and skills
Payments	Service and unit based	Population/capitation based contracting
Economic Discipline	Payment controls and shifting of responsibilities	Balanced incentives, roles and responsibilities, with economic predictability
		Accountability and collaboration
Quality	Episodic and retrospective evaluation	Continuous quality improvement and outcomes orientation
	Patient focus	Holistic and quality of life focus
Organization and Delivery	Individualized market arrangements, segmentation and horizontal competition	Vertically integrated, community-based networks focusing on health status, prevention, quality and collaboration

ty of people stay in a capitated plan when they reach 65 and qualify for Medicare. Other areas of the nation are experimenting with similar enrollment shifts, albeit in smaller numbers.

It is essential that the destructive concept, that quality is synonymous with quantity in health care, be erased from the public's mind. As the delivery system evolves into integrated networks, value will be based on a balance of outcomes—medically, socially, and economically.

PROVIDER INTERDEPENDENCE

A nationwide uniform benefit package will define the basic services which are available to everyone. Each network must be broad enough in scope and expertise to provide the services. By necessity, then, the networks will encompass a large number of providers.

This integration is vital because under the current system, providers are isolated, independent, and generally behave in a mutually exclusive manner. This is the antithesis of modern business concepts, which stress common vision and values, teamwork, and communication as essential to winning organizations. Like any successful business, community health networks must be team-oriented with individual accountability. All providers within a community health network must have clear vision, qualitative measures, common goals, congruent motivations, and an interdependent esprit de corps to succeed. Empowerment of employees within an organization is analogous to joint empowerment of providers within a community health network. Health care will achieve quality and cost containment only when it is in the individual provider's interest to work in a way that serves the common good.

The idea that providers bear the responsibility for improving health status is incompatible with a curative-oriented system and conflicts with the inherent human motivations. Only when providers are given the responsibility for health status, in a competitive arena where it is in their interest to efficiently produce high-quality services at the lowest possible price, will the vision be achieved. With a fixed amount of money available annually to the community health network through capitation, providers will have the strong incentive to become more efficient in their allocation of resources and provision of service.

INDIVIDUAL COMPETITION HAS FAILED

Some fee-for-service proponents claim that individual competition is working to hold down prices. They argue that free-market forces are at work in the present system, offering as proof the fact that their unit costs and charges are less than some other providers'. While they may indeed provide individual units of service at lower charges than the others in the community, the argument ultimately fails because this type of horizontal competition increases the number of services available, total utilization and thus the total cost of services nationwide. For example, if there is adequate capacity in the system, adding new providers who charge less per unit of service will not lower the total costs expended. It simply creates a new provider layer that, in the long run, actually adds to the expansion of services and technology, higher utilization, and increased costs.

ALIGNING INCENTIVES

The foundation of the new delivery system is a new set of incentives that serve to modify the behavior of everyone within the health care equation. The individuals who use the system, while maintaining choice of community health networks, will be required to act more responsibly regarding their health and consumption of health care resources. Those who finance the system will no longer be burdened with workers' compensation problems, or exclusionary rulings by third-party carriers. The carriers themselves will be freed from the tremendous expense of audit and utilization reviews.

The government's role will be modified to that of participant and facilitator, instead of a command-and-control agent. This cops-and-robbers scenario, which has preoccupied providers with trying to live within the system and out-maneuver the control agents, will give way to a cooperative and far more efficient and satisfactory relationship.

PREVENTATIVE MEDICINE EMPHASIS

These new incentives will generate powerful and positive changes in the way health care is delivered. For example, preventative medicine, which historically has received mostly lip service in the past, will likely be fully embraced by the community health network. Currently, there is little financial incentive for providers to emphasize prevention, especially in comparison to the financial rewards of focusing on episodic intervention. As a result, preventative medicine has been relegated to the fringes of the medical world. Historically, the vast bulk of research and development funds, exclusive of public health, have been allocated to the creation of new diagnostic and therapeutic technologies and procedures. Prestige has been built on the exotic and costly side of health care.

For the first time, all providers will be better off keeping patients healthy than with treating sick ones. Naturally, a shift toward emphasizing preventative medicine will take place. It is likely that more importance will be placed on educating patients about living healthy lifestyles, along with a corresponding shift in research and development funding for preventative disciplines. Incentive payments to community health networks that improve health status would add to the likelihood of prevention and health promotion.

This shift will help create a powerful partnership between providers and patients and will improve health standards nationwide. People will be encouraged through education and provider influence to play a more active role in their health-related and life-style choices.

This heightened awareness is likely to have a significant ripple effect toward increasing our quality of life. It should lead to a heightened awareness of the environmental factors that affect our health, such as the quality of air, water, food, and so on. Increased understanding of how these issues affect our health will ultimately translate to better individual choices.

How we prevent diseases and costly therapeutic intervention is important in the overall goal of moving toward affordable and accessible health care. An emphasis on screening and prevention, primary care and consultation, ambulatory alternatives, and a preference for low-tech services when appropriate is essential. The potential exists for the community health networks to play an exciting new role in the development of educational, training, and research programs that emphasize prevention.

ACHIEVING UNIVERSAL ACCESS

Universal access is the backbone of the new paradigm. Without universal coverage, the other components of reform fall apart. If every resident has a health card backed by guaranteed payment, regional networks' competitiveness will generate breakthroughs that allow the system to achieve universal access to health care. Internal collaboration becomes a natural, and community health network competition is transformed to an unprecedented level of progressive competition.

TOWARD AN AFFORDABLE SYSTEM

The challenge to each community health network is to
arrange for the best distribution of necessary providers
and resources so that the uniform benefit package can be
delivered and the health care status of all enrolled persons
can be improved. Within each network, the self-governing
providers must decide how they will deploy resources and
divide the capitated payment revenues. The entire thrust
of the integrated network is toward improving individual
health care in a cost-effective manner so it can compete
with the other networks.

A basic element in cost containment within the
community health networks is the role of generalist doctors. Physician distribution and specialization are two factors that dramatically impact health care costs. When
individuals have unlimited access to specialists, without
the financial accountability of paying directly for such
choices, the temptation to overuse the system is great.
People bypass generalists in favor of specialists, based on
the perceived concept that when it comes to their own
health, they need a specialist. This creates a self-fulfilling
prophecy that more and more specialists are needed. The
referral patterns among physicians and the high use of
consultations add to the utilization-demand cycle.

PRIMARY CARE GATEKEEPERS

Managing the consumption of specialized services is vital
to holding down costs. The new paradigm calls for internal controls within the community health networks by
establishing generalist physicians as the "gatekeepers" for
patients. While primary-care is not an island in itself, it is
the essential medical cornerstone of the network. A base

of generalist practitioners holds the best opportunity for maintaining the proper use of specialized resources. It propels the relatively low cost providers to the forefront of the system, while preventing the overutilization of high-cost specialty care. The gatekeepers' obligation is to keep enrollees healthy and to refer patients to high-tech, specialty services when necessary.

Traditionally, generalist physicians have not enjoyed the reputation of more highly compensated specialists. A key to successful community health networks is their ability to place generalists in the high-tech mainstream while keeping their focus on nonhospital practice. This shift will affect their relationship with specialists and is a challenge to manage because of the shifts in political influence and compensation.

THE ESSENTIAL LINKS

The link between the capitated financing system and integrated delivery network is crucial. Some have called for integrated networks without a capitation or bundled payment system. This will be less effective because it does not necessarily align the motivation and incentives of the providers. Without a finite and predictable amount of money going into the networks, the providers will be motivated, even within networks, to spar with government and payers to preserve the status quo.

Each of the components outlined in this book are interdependent and are vital to the success of the new paradigm. Subtract any one of them from the equation and the entire structure is greatly weakened. Without the employer-sponsored financing system, for example, the effort would falter because universal access is less likely to occur. Absent the underwriting reforms, third-party exclusionary rules will continue to multiply as insurance carriers scramble to rid themselves of "risky" clients. Without all of the reforms, the do-more-to-make-more incentive will not be replaced with incentives for collaboration among providers within a network. Without this crucial motivational change, there will be no corresponding reduction in the duplication of services and technology. Further, limited practice health professionals will have no reason to become part of an integrated network.

Similarly, subtracting either the finance or the payment components from the model will force insurance companies and other third-party carriers to continue their costly systems of external audit and utilization reviews and predatory exclusionary practices. Without the formation of competing integrated delivery networks in urbanized areas, less meaningful long-term reform will be accomplished. As long as providers are encouraged to duplicate services and technology, no real cost controls can be achieved.

If, through the lack of political will or social courage, any one of these elements is lacking, we will be forced by the continuing rise in health care costs to reverse course toward the other option—governmental control.

DEFINING THE NETWORKS

Successful delivery networks will be the major component of community health networks. By necessity, they will be customer-oriented and dedicated to achieving a deep understanding of the needs and preferences of the regional populations they serve. They will be community-based, accessible, and responsive in ways that are not possible when providers operate as separate, competing entities.

For example, deployment of providers and resources will conform to community needs. Convenient sites will be located close to population clusters or primary work areas. Access to primary care, referrals for specialty care, and ancillary services will be more efficient.

All these services will be coordinated within a single network, so patients and providers can focus on patients rather than trying to adhere to administrative procedures and jumping through hoops to justify every service. The ability of networks to focus on regional populations in defined geographic areas fosters more accurate diagnosis and care, while specialty care can be concentrated for best results. The service itself will be provided in a more timely and friendly manner because patient satisfaction, quality and outcomes will be the driving market force. Individual providers will no longer be in a position to dictate service standards to patients or independently order services without considering other factors.

At the same time, the economies of scale achieved by the networks allow for appropriate acquisition of new technologies and training of new health professionals. This also means lower debt-service costs, and thus greater financial stability and predictability.

SELF-DIRECTED NETWORKS

Other significant elements in the success of each network include flexibility and autonomy. Each network must be self-designed to meet the needs of the community; it is unlikely that any two networks will be exactly the same. Networks must provide all the services required under the uniform benefit package, but for the most part their internal structures, including allocation of finances, will be determined by their members. This freedom allows each community health network to adapt itself to whatever design best meets the needs of the community it serves.

While all community health networks will receive funding through capitation payments, it will be up to the providers within the network to determine the method of payment to network participants. For example, physicians could be paid on a fee schedule, salary, capitated rate, or other basis. Hospitals could be paid on the basis of costs, prospective rates, per admission or other unit of service, capitated rates, global budgets, or other factors.

For bottom-up negotiations to produce economic predictability, a negotiating arm must be established to purchase coverage from community health networks. Individuals and businesses with fewer than 100 employees, who lack the buying power or resources to negotiate with community health networks, must rely on collective representation to arrange coverage options for them. States, through a single negotiating body, or through regional purchasing pools, should designate the purchasing regions. Regional negotiating bodies are called health alliances. They could be public in nature, quasi-public or not-for-profit private organizations.

Health alliances would negotiate capitation rates for the uniform benefit package with community health networks. Individuals could choose the community health network they prefer, paying a higher amount if they select a higher cost community health network. Employers would pay the same amount for every employee, in the range of 75 to 80 percent of the capitated premium. This dynamic creates pressure on community health networks to be competitively priced, thereby producing market-driven economic discipline from the best source—local communities.

PUBLIC ACCOUNTABILITY

Community health networks should have the right to self-determination without government attempting to micro-manage their internal affairs. However, community health networks must be accountable to all stakeholders for their performance on an on-going basis.

This public accountability promotes two positive results: First, it securely links providers and patients to a common goal—to improve health status and provide quality health care at a reasonable cost. Second, it furnishes individuals with the data and information to use when choosing a community health network. The accountability can be achieved through governmental agencies and alliances. Regular reports would be available to the community on the community health networks' performance in patient satisfaction, outcomes, progress in health status, cost, and financial viability. The results could be reported by government through media outlets on a regular basis, with specific information provided to the public by alliances prior to open-enrollment periods. This would allow policy makers, alliances, and individuals the opportunity to scrutinize and compare community health networks.

PROVIDERS MUST SUPPORT CHANGE

The major provider groups, including physicians and hospitals, have a unique opportunity to play a major role in the restructuring of the health care delivery system. Many will enthusiastically support the change, and some will resist it. Because disruption in the status quo will occur, many providers will feel threatened. There is little doubt that the professionals involved with the delivery of health care services have the intelligence and ingenuity to make the change. However, they must be encouraged to do so through a groundswell of public support and the backing of wise and clear-sighted public policy. Similarly, public officials are likely to make the tough decisions about financing and payment systems only when convinced that strong public support exists. Once this hurdle is cleared, reform of the delivery system will follow.

A word of caution is in order. Not all providers, or provider groups, may survive. In fact, if there is no change in the number of providers and types of providers, the maximum results from reform will not be achieved. As painful as it is, the reality of resizing is as crucial for providers as it is for carriers, government, and patients.

THE UNIFORM BENEFIT PACKAGE

The uniform benefit package should define basic health services for its members, as needed and without time or cost limitations. A starting point follows:

1) Physician services
2) Medically necessary physical and mental inpatient hospital services.
3) Medically necessary physical and mental outpatient services.
4) Home health services provided in a noninstitutional setting at a member's home by health care personnel, as prescribed or directed by the responsible physician or other authority designated by the community health network.

5) Nursing facility care for at least thirty days per episode of illness, with a maximum of sixty days per year.
6) Preventive health services, which shall be made available to members and include at least the following:

- Voluntary family planning services
- Infertility services
- Prenatal care
- Well-child care from birth
- Periodic health evaluations for adults as determined by the community health network
- Eye and ear examinations for children through age seventeen, to determine the need for vision and hearing correction
- Pediatric and adult immunizations, in accord with accepted medical practices
- Basic dental services for children under six years of age
- Other health services that are not included in the uniform benefit package (may be limited in time and cost)

7) Prescription drugs and medicines (could be made available only in capitated arrangements to encourage enrollment into the economically predictable plans)
8) To the extent that a natural disaster, war, riot, civil insurrection, epidemic or any other emergency or similar event not within the control of a community health network results in the facilities, personnel or financial resources of a network being unavailable to provide or arrange for the provision of the uniform benefit package, the community health network is

required only to make a good-faith effort to provide or arrange for the provision of the service, taking into account the impact of the event. An event is not within the control of a community health network if it cannot exercise influence or dominion over its occurrence.

9) Instructions to the community health networks' members on procedures to be followed to secure medically necessary emergency health services, both in the service area and out of the service area.

The following would not be required services in the uniform benefit package (although they could be provided at the option of the community health network):

1) Cosmetic appliances and artificial aids
2) Cosmetic surgery, unless medically necessary
3) Nonprescribed or over-the-counter drugs and medicines
4) Ambulance services, unless medically necessary
5) Care for military service-connected disabilities for which the member is legally entitled to services provided by the military and for which facilities are reasonably available
6) Care for conditions that state or local law requires be treated in a public facility
7) Dental services for persons six years of age or older
8) Custodial or domiciliary institutional care
9) Experimental medical, surgical, or other health care procedures, unless approved by the policy-making body of the community health network
10) Unusual and infrequently provided health services that are not necessary for the protection of individual health.

Community health networks should be allowed to apply deductibles and co-payments within limits that are established by the National Health Board. Such out-of-pocket expenditures should be directed to: promoting health and judicious use of health resources, relying on the person's own community health network for services and instilling personal responsibility into the attitude of every American.

Further, higher out-of-pocket expenditures should be permitted when enrolled persons select more costly options, higher priced community health networks and independent providers.

NEW ROLES FOR HEALTH PROVIDERS

It would be comforting to think that health providers' roles evolved in a well-designed and meaningful way. After all, these professionals render one of society's most important services. Unfortunately, regressive incentives and short-sighted policies have encouraged fragmentation, duplication, and greater utilization—all of which result in higher costs.

The evolution of provider roles has been shaped more by happenstance and political ricochet than by a public health policy and strategic planning. Consider the years following World War II, when federal money flowed into new hospitals, medical schools and research, increasing the number of physicians and hospitals and promoting research and development projects and technological advancements. The effect of this well-intentioned effort was to drastically alter the entire medical-industrial complex.

The influx of money and prestige attracted thousands of would-be doctors to medical schools around the country. Specialization was encouraged. Jurisdictional disputes and turf wars began to emerge resulting in stratification and the duplication of technology and efforts, fueling rising costs and the need for greater compensation from patients and third-party payers. The proliferation and specialization led to an expansion of licensing and certification, especially for those who dealt directly with the public, for example, physicians, dentists, clinical psychologists, nurses and pharmacists. Licensing, certification and registration became not only ways of establishing standards and qualifications, they paved the way for providers to gain a franchise. Those not directly accessible to the public— therapists, technicians, and lab analysts—also began to scramble to secure licensure and solidify their positions and raise the financial value of their services.

In fairness to the providers, this quixotic dilemma was not created so much by doctors or hospitals as by the fact that the government has not yet recognized that health care is a unique industry. More than 70 percent of the population believes health care is a right, and 70 percent will not agree to pay higher taxes to achieve the goal.

Governmental overpromising and underfunding result. We must change the way that government thinks about health and providers.

GENERALIST PHYSICIAN IN CONTROL

The roles of providers within the networks will elicit a subtle, but substantial change. Generalist physicians should be the entry point into the network. The gatekeeper's primary responsibility will be to promote wellness, check and interview each patient (except emergency patients), and treat or refer them to the appropriate provider. If the generalist is assisted by a nonphysician, such as a nurse practitioner, protocols and patient satisfaction will ensure quality and continuity of care.

On the whole, more medical students should be directed toward providing general and preventative medicine, through governmental funding incentives, community health network support and public demand. A vital change within the new system will be that specialists, who provide the most expensive care and now account for more than 60 percent of all physicians, will no longer dominate. The new paradigm reverses that trend.

Here's how it will work: When Uncle Harry suffers from a stomach disorder, he goes to his provider network. He is certain he has an ulcer and requests to see a stomach specialist right away. First, he is screened and tested by a generalist physician, the gatekeeper, who finds that he does not have an ulcer but has eaten too many hot peppers. Uncle Harry is given some antiacid tablets, dietary advice, and an exercise regimen. His problem is solved without a costly visit to a specialist, or a series of expensive and unnecessary tests.

One of the obstacles that must be overcome is the public's current perception that only specialists can solve certain medical problems. As a nation, we have fallen into the habit of diagnosing our own ailments, and immediately turning to specialists for help. We must reverse this pattern and reestablish trust in primary care. Specialists will still be there if we need them, but this system will ensure that we need them before we utilize them.

Community health networks will educate their enrollees to seek care through the system. Otherwise, the cost to the community health network will be higher and the patient will incur greater out-of-pocket expense. These important financial incentives will help decrease unwarranted patient demands.

COORDINATED CARE

Within an integrated network, the providers will find their roles radically altered since they must communicate, coordinate care, and fully cooperate with each other to prosper. Unlike the current system, in which each provider must compete against every other, the new system will require teamwork and trust.

Developing these new skills may take time because they have not been required of providers outside risk bearing organizations. But given the correct incentives, it is likely a new model of physician will emerge, one who practices efficient team medicine. A new culture is necessary, one that makes teamwork, communications and coordination the foundation of quality and professional reward.

Competition between provider networks—not between the individual providers within a network—will keep the networks lean, avoiding unnecessary duplication of personnel or technology. It will not benefit an individual provider to try to take advantage of the providers in the network because if the group fails, the individual provider can't succeed.

The driving force behind this new system—the source of its power—is the newly created environment of economic discipline. For the first time in the history of health care, it will provide a symbiotic dynamic whereby providers' goals are aligned with the carriers', public's and patients' goals. One single reality overrides all others—the system that delivers quality service efficiently and keeps its patients the healthiest will be the most successful.

MUTUAL TRUST

Good communication and mutual respect must exist among the generalists, specialists, and other providers. If an individual provider loses that respect because of poor or excessive practices, he or she will be eliminated from that network. The providers within the network can't keep colleagues they don't trust, who fail to deliver efficient, high-quality care, or who attempt to take advantage of the network. It is in the gatekeeper's best interest to refer patients to competent specialists, who will treat them with skill and respect. Conversely, the specialist must trust the primary-care physician to make the correct diagnosis and referrals.

On the other hand, physicians also serve as advocates for their patients and this responsibility must be balanced with cost considerations and quality. To prevent under-utilization and inadequate care, the ultimate responsibility for practice protocols and quality must rest with a doctor's peers, thereby preserving the clinical quality and appropriateness of care.

CHECKS AND BALANCES

Several checks and balances are built into the new system, both for the patients and the providers. First, patients would be entitled to a second opinion, at the gatekeeper and referral stages. If they are still dissatisfied with the second opinion, they have the freedom to appeal or to circumvent the gatekeeper and go outside the network to see a specialist on a private basis. However, patients must pay for all or a substantial portion of that service out of their own pockets. This economic discipline is essential to the success of a system built on finite resources. Patients will pay for their unauthorized use of services, providing a self-governing discipline for themselves as well as providers.

Second, a 12-month, renewable enrollment contract will protect consumers and assure them the choice of networks and providers that offer the highest quality service at the best prices. The third check is the provision that state governments monitor the performances of the provider networks. This can be done like the way that many states currently monitor health insurance companies, health maintenance organizations, and health providers. These performance appraisals, which include consumer satisfaction and complaints (from grievances to legal filings) are logged and reported annually or semiannually. The results would be released to the media, which usually consider them headline news. Armed with this information, their own personal experiences, and com-

parative reports published annually, groups and consumers will be able to make wise choices regarding
provider networks.

In addition, each person will receive a report card of
the community health networks in his or her area prior to
the annual enrollment date. This comparative data report
will arm each individual with the information to make a
more informed choice in selecting a community health
network. The questionable payer and provider organizations—some of which have grown fat on the inequities of
the present system—will not be able to withstand the heat
of that kind of scrutiny. The result will be that only the
strongest and best provider networks will survive and
flourish. There will be no room for cherry pickers, chisel-
ers, fat-cats, or speculators in the new system.

The fourth check on the system will arise from the
providers' personal value systems. This, of course, exists
now, because the vast majority of health providers and
institutions have a strong sense of their mission to treat
patients with dignity and respect.

The new system will bring all surgical and other procedures into sharper focus since networks will no longer
directly profit from each individual procedure. As a result,
a drastic drop in the number of diagnostic tests, surgeries,
and other procedures can be expected.

Another check on the system for consumers is the
entire cloud of malpractice liability. The right of patients
to sue doctors, hospitals and others suspected of malpractice will remain a powerful deterrent to inadequate practices or negligence. Left unchecked, however, plaintiff
attorneys can take advantage of the system. To curtail
such litigiousness and reduce the pressures to practice
defensively, minimum tort reforms (outlined in chapter 8)
are needed.

The number of malpractice suits may decrease under the new system as the goals of the providers and patients become better aligned. Keeping patients well and away from overuse of expensive technology will be a mutual goal of everybody involved in the network. Moreover, the self-governing measures within the networks will help curb poor medical practices.

Hospital claim allegations by location*
United States: 1990-1992

Location/Allegations	Number of Claims			% of Total Claims			Average Cost		
	1990	1991	1992	1990	1991	1992	1990	1991	1992
Patient Care Area	1,989	1,972	1,890	31.1%	30.4%	29.2%	$36,634	$41,603	$47,809
Emergency Department	1,214	1,208	1,215	19.0	18.7	19.0	40,006	45,101	40,741
Inpatient Surgery	1,091	1,098	1,115	17.0	16.9	17.2	34,731	40,799	39,360
Obstetrical Care	706	755	775	11.0	11.7	12.0	99,155	94,620	96,940
Outpatient Services	260	285	278	4.1	4.4	4.3	21,665	26,577	22,911
Outpatient Surgery	186	205	231	2.9	3.2	3.5	17,462	25,293	49,088
Psychiatric Care	191	218	228	3.0	3.4	3.5	41,739	39,969	26,820
Radiological Services	231	203	205	3.6	3.1	3.2	21,768	26,662	31,309
Therapy Services	16	17	20	0.2	0.3	0.3	8,411	28,916	27,281
Other Areas	518	509	501	8.1	7.9	7.8	40,180	33,058	23,899

* All claims reported by St. Paul insured hospitals representing approximately one quarter of the nation's hospitals.

SOURCE: St. Paul Marine and Fire Insurance Company, *Update, Hospitals*, "The St. Paul's 1991-1993 Annual Report to Policyholders," St. Paul, 1991-1993.

A final check is the anti-trust laws. Relief is necessary from the Federal Trade Commission's and Department of Justice's roadblocks to sharing services, technology, and facilities. Providers and networks can not operate under the historic rules. On September 15, 1993, federal antitrust guidelines were released, which opened the door for collaborative activities.

MEDICAL CATCH-22

The alignment of patient and provider goals is critical. The opposite exists today and providers are stuck in a philosophical Catch-22. Imagine what would happen to health providers if all their patients suddenly became healthy. The system would fall apart.

We have put our health providers in an absurd position. They pledge to help heal the sick and injured, yet total success would mean bankruptcy. On one hand, we ask them to heal the sick and lower costs, but on the other we have structured their economics in the opposite direction. Little wonder the system is on the brink of a meltdown.

PROVIDERS LEAD PREVENTION

Certainly, preventative health practices are a shared responsibility between patient and physician, but physicians should lead the way. Preventative medicine has largely been relegated to the Public Health Service, states and local governments. Most important, third-party carriers shun payments for many preventative efforts. In recent years, public health funding through governmental programs has fallen victim to the budget-cutting knife, creating a crisis for the public, especially for vulnerable populations.

The damage done by this inconsistency is enormous, both in financial and human terms. Implementing prevention measures, such as educating patients on diet, how to reduce stress, smoking, and proper exercise habits, have a minuscule cost compared to the cost of intervention.

The treatment of heart disease, the leading cause of premature death in the U.S. is perhaps the best example. More than 700,000 Americans die annually from coronary heart disease; and of these, 262,000 will die before they reach a hospital. This is despite the fact that in 1991, some 407,000 coronary-artery bypass grafts were performed at an average cost of $35,000 apiece. The American Heart Association estimates that nearly $110 billion was spent on cardiovascular diseases in 1991. Yet, relatively little of that was spent on preventative measures for the people who are not yet acutely affected. Without changing the incentives within the present system, we are doomed to continue spending exorbitant amounts on intervention, without a corresponding increase in the nation's health status.

Heart disease data
United States: Select Years 1973-1990

Year	Heart Disease Deaths	Rate Per 100,000 Population	Percent Of Total Deaths
1973	757,075	360.8	38.4%
1975	716,215	338.9	37.8
1980	763,060	343.0	38.4
1985	775,890	325.0	37.2
1990	720,058	289.5	33.5
1991*	718,090	283.3	33.2

* Provisional Data

SOURCE:National Center for Health Statistics, *Vital Statistics of the United States*, 1973 and 1975, Volume II, Mortality, Parts A and B, 1975 and 1977. National Center for Health Statistics, *Monthly Vital Statistics Report*, "Annual Summary, Birth, Deaths, Marriages: US, 1980, 1985 and 1990," Vol. 40 #13, 1981-1993, Hyattsville. National Center for Health Statistics, *Monthly Vital Statistics*, "Advance Report of Final Mortality," Vol. 41 #7, Hyattsville, 1993.

Under the new paradigm, preventative medicine will come out of the closet and move to the forefront of provider practice. It will assume a much higher profile at medical education institutions, and its evolution should

Cardiovascular disease costs*

United States: 1988-1993 (000)

Year	Dollars	Percent Annual Change
1988	$88,700,000	. .
1989	88,200,000	-0.6%
1990	94,500,000	7.1
1991	101,300,000	7.2
1992	108,900,000	7.5
1993†	117,400,000	7.8

* Includes cost of physician and nursing services, hospital and nursing home services, medications and lost productivity resulting from disability.
† Projected.

SOURCE: American Heart Association, *1988-1993 Heart and Stroke Facts*, 1988-1993, Dallas.

increase at an accelerated rate. This emphasis on prevention should provide for a healthier society over time and,
thus, a decrease in total health expenditures.

PHYSICIAN ACCEPTANCE

There is a perception that doctors will resist joining delivery networks because they favor individual autonomy.
Growing evidence indicates that the opposite is true, that
physicians are steering away from hanging out individual
shingles in favor of multi-specialty groups and other collaborative settings. As an example, a recent graduating
class of pediatricians from a University of California resi-
dency program chose to become affiliated with integrated
systems or multi-specialty groups. It wasn't important for
them to open independent offices. Clinical autonomy and
financial independence—two key desires of most individual practitioners—are still present in truly integrated
delivery networks.

Most young physicians cannot afford all the things
they need for an individual, independent practice without

placing themselves deeper into debt. A reasonably
equipped office could include an X-ray unit, a small lab,
testing equipment, space to treat patients, a sophisticated
computer system that handles billing and payroll, and a
variety of other technological products. Staff would also
be needed—usually amounting to a bookkeeper, recep-
tionist, and at least one nurse professional. All of this is
expensive and inefficient. The typical independent physician takes home less than 60 percent of the payments he
or she receives. The inefficiency of this approach becomes
apparent.

Average self-employed physician professional expenses

United States: 1979 and 1991 (000)

Physician Specialty	Average Professional Expenses*	
	1979	1991
General Practice	$ 55.7	$ 146.4
Internal Medicine	52.5	159.0
Surgery	69.3	215.6
Pediatrics	51.0	145.4
Obstetrics/Gynecology	67.0	236.2
Radiology	51.0	194.2
Psychiatry	23.1	62.6
Anesthesiology	26.3	115.9
Pathology	N/A	149.1
All Physicians	**52.9**	**168.4**

* Professional expenses include non-physician payroll, professional insurance, medical
  equipment, and office expenses.

SOURCE: California Medical Association, *Physicians and Health Care Statistics,* 1981,
San Francisco. American Medical Association, *Socioeconomic Characteristics of Medical Practice,*
1993, Chicago.

Networks offer other benefits to physicians. Administration costs can be lower. Utilities and other costs are
shared. More professional support exists and, therefore,
the quality of care usually rises. Immediate referrals to
appropriate practitioners can be made, making it more

convenient for patients. Doctors will do less paperwork and more practice. As single practitioners, many physicians find themselves stretched to the breaking point. In addition to treating patients, they must be administrators, personnel managers, business people, entrepreneurs, technical experts, and tenants or landlords. They will practice medicine successfully only if they master these other skills. The distractions are too much for many physicians. They find that working within a network provides them the freedom to pursue their primary objective—the practice of high-quality medicine.

HOSPITAL'S ROLE

Hospitals will continue to provide the traditional acute care and support services, but their role must change. They will no longer be a separate entity. They will become part of an integrated network, providing the special services required in the uniform benefit package.

One of the biggest differences will be how hospitals are utilized. Currently, it costs physicians little to utilize expensive hospital resources. In the new system, it will be in the doctors' collective interest to utilize the hospital only when it actually produces the right or best results.

The effect will be a different motivation for deploying and consuming hospital resources. The objective will not be doing more to make more or competing to see who can build the largest hospital or offer the most services, but rather determining the most economical way of providing high-quality acute and episodic care.

Currently, hospitals are under-utilized and many are suffering financial stress. Thus, the economic impulse is to find some way to recover by filling the empty beds. This will change under the new system because there will be no economic incentive to expand hospital capacity or utilize resources for financial gain. Hospitals will be cost centers within a network rather than generators of revenue. Consequently, the number of available beds is likely to drop and the capacity of hospitals will be reduced or used differently. A certain floor of a hospital may provide a totally different service for the network. Some hospitals may be closed or replaced with alternative facilities for the patients' convenience. Others, especially larger hospitals, probably will become intensive care-oriented centers, providing the most expensive acute-care services.

Collectively, hospitals within a delivery network will compete with the hospitals in other provider networks. They will also join forces with the other providers in their own networks to form a team that competitively delivers the uniform benefit package.

The end result will be that most hospitals will become smaller, leaner, and more efficient. All hospital services will still be available, but only for those who really require them.

SPECIAL CIRCUMSTANCES

It may be necessary for a hospital to contract with more than one network. This is especially true for specialty facilities and services, such as burn and trauma centers, transplant facilities, children's hospitals, rehabilitation facilities, mental health, teaching, and other specialty hospitals.

It may not make economic sense for each network to have its own specialty hospital, teaching institution, burn unit, or trauma center because the network probably couldn't staff or afford it. The facilities wouldn't be used enough to justify it. However, by contracting out to several networks, these special facilities will gain the necessary volume to provide efficient, high-quality services.

The same concept applies to medical education programs. Medical education must survive to ensure a continuing supply of physicians and other professionals and the system must provide some financial support for medical education. Currently, part of this cost is built into the teaching hospital's charges. Federal support should be continued to ensure the viability of educational programs. A portion of premiums paid from employers and government should be set aside to ensure adequate funding for medical education.

The channeling of a portion of the research dollars to community health networks will likewise improve the quality, focus, and resources devoted to experimentation and research. Today, the allocation of research funds is not always focused on the nation's highest public health priorities. For reform to be effective, all aspects of the system, including research, must share a common vision.

GEOGRAPHICAL CHANGES

It is a given that the number of providers, and sites at which they operate, will change dramatically under the new system. There will be fewer independent doctors' offices, hospitals, and other provider sites.

At first glance, this may seem an alarming trend. Won't fewer provider outlets translate into a decrease in service? The answer is no! While the outlets may decrease in number, service will actually increase in quality and accessibility. Currently, providers are located in areas for many reasons. A doctor may have chosen the site because it was close to his or her home, because he or she got a good deal on the building or rental lease, or because it made sense given the traditional incentives.

But under the new system, there will only be one reason for a network to locate an office or service in a given location—because it is cost-effective, quality enhancing, and a convenient site for the patients. There will be too much at stake for the network to use any other reason for selecting delivery sites.

The geographical look of the new system will undoubtedly be different than it is today. Except in rural areas, there will be few single-provider offices. The doctor's office will even change inside. The use of new technologies, integration with other network locations, and streamlining will make the legendary wait in the doctor's office more manageable. Physicians, under pressure to provide the highest quality service, will be motivated to eliminate this irritant. Videocommunications, home care, and a variety of other technologies will be utilized to help decrease the need for office visits.

The key to the reorganization is that the community health network has a strong incentive to deploy resources where they will most efficiently serve that network's customers. The bottom line is, if it doesn't meet the standards and desires of patients, the network will fail. Ultimately, people will be better served.

CHANGE IN PHARMACIES

Similarly, pharmacies will probably drop in number as they compete for a place in the community health networks. Those that cannot or will not provide top quality service at the lowest possible prices will fail. The result will be a streamlined pharmaceutical distribution industry. Strategically placed outlets will likely remain near doctors' offices and other locations where they are most accessible.

Some important changes will take place internally. Pharmacies, as essential members of the network, will also be under pressure to keep prices of covered drugs down. Community health networks will pressure drug manufacturers to keep costs in line. Use of generic drugs will increase. The end result will be better market-control of the cost of prescription drugs.

PATIENT ACCOUNTABILITY

Just as the roles of the providers change, so does the role of patients. They will be oriented through financial consequences and education on how to use the system. They will be given the responsibility to use it correctly. Penalties will exist for using services in an irresponsible manner. For instance, if a patient has a headache and opts to be treated in the trauma center against the recommendation of the gatekeeper, the cost won't be covered and the patient must foot all or a significant portion of the bill. Thus, providers and patients equally share the responsibility for using the network properly. Applied universally to all patients and providers, significant changes in behavior will close the gap between real needs and disjointed expectations.

THE BOTTOM LINE—QUALITY

This changing of roles will not lead to the denigration of health care. In fact, the opposite will be true as the economic pivot point of the system becomes the patient's health status. It means the old way of doing business, the costly horizontal expansion of technology and delivery, goes the way of the Edsel. It will be replaced by networks of providers in new roles working together toward a single goal—improved health status and top-quality health care.

THE NEW ORDER

▼

Health care does not exist within a vacuum. It is an essential part of the fabric of society. Simple legislation won't reform the system, nor will cosmetic or superficial changes. Long-term change will require shifts in public and private accountability, attitudes, and policies. Only deep-rooted reform that alters the incentives of every stakeholder is sufficient to meet the challenge and modify the behavior of providers, consumers, government, and payers of health care services.

Piecemeal public policy and private practices have created todays' perverse incentives and allowed the economic consequences to be masked. In essence, we have created the problem ourselves. Attempts to control it through governmental underfunding, cutting payments, shifting costs, private contracting and other isolated efforts have failed. Health care must take on a new dimension. It must be viewed as a whole, as an integrated part of society and our personal lives, rather than an episodic experience for providers and patients. It must be more than an isolated system where people recover from illness or injury, then return to the old way of doing things. Health and well-being must become an integral part of society, based on attitudes, habits, policies, and expectations.

BUILDING A COMMON VISION

If we intend to bring economic discipline to a diverse, multicultural society, then we must bring together a newly aligned vision of health, supported by all those who can affect the outcome.

Much can be said about the breakdown of family values and the family unit, the rising incidence of violence, and the destructive practices of individuals. All of these are underlying societal problems that affect health care. They must be addressed, with the highest priority assigned to relying on the family as the foundation of our society.

Other components of life that impact attitudes and behavior must share responsibility. The educational and health care systems, government, media, entertainment industry, and business community must all buy into the concept of health and well-being as an individual responsibility.

If health becomes a community affair, if it becomes a responsibility of everyone—and not just everyone else— then we have the opportunity to refocus on health and improve health status. This emphasis has become lost through the emergence of insurance and other policies that prevent people from taking responsibility for their health. The right to life, liberty, and the pursuit of happiness inherently depends upon a healthy society.

In the last thirty years, government has given much lip service to the idea that health care is a right. However, many of the policy practices it has established are contrary to that concept.

For instance, the government stresses the need to keep health care costs down, but in many cases does nothing to aid in achieving that goal. In hospitals across the nation, patients who do not have health care are increasingly using hospital emergency rooms to obtain their primary care services. Under these circumstances, it is impossible to decrease costs.

One city's hospitals came up with a much more economical and sensible way of treating these patients. The hospitals created a Care Van that visited communities where most of these patients resided. The Care Van went to the neighborhoods one or two evenings a week to provide routine health care and educate the people on preventative practices. Consequently, the misuse of emergency room services decreased and the community's overall health care status improved. The success of the Care Van illustrates how theory and practice must support one another.

Significant social progress is possible only when public policies are aligned with the initiatives and efforts of the private sector. Government mandates alone, especially ones that run counter to the defined mission, do not work.

The vision that every resident of the U.S. is entitled to equitable access to wellness through health care is integral. That vision for quality health care must include physical and mental health care, and services for the abuse of chemical substances.

In order to achieve an optimally healthy society, a viable health care infrastructure is needed. The infrastructure must reflect economic discipline and predictability. It must also be consistent with the vision of improving health status through education, the promotion of preventative practices and wellness, and with the delivery of coordinated and appropriate services in a cost-effective manner.

Under the new order, health care must be based on the concept that it is a service that must be available to everyone; it must exemplify the highest human element and spirit. Dignity must extend beyond individuals or groups, to be fully realized only when health care is accessible to everyone in society. The value of life depends on how we manage life, how we manage health, and how we manage the dying process.

MIND, BODY AND SOUL

In the new order, health care must be viewed jointly as an individual and a societal responsibility. Both sides of this equation must provide leadership based on a common vision, shared goals, and mutually agreeable ways to reach those goals.

This leadership is essential to blaze the way toward public acceptance of the new financing, payment, and delivery aspects of health care.

While the government, providers, carriers, and the media can play key roles in communicating the major elements of the new health care plan, much of the opportunity lies within the schools. The educational curriculum of kindergarten through high school must be altered to build a working knowledge of the importance of health, preventive practices, and health services. Otherwise, there is a disconnection between a healthy mind that achieves academic success and physical and mental health. These three elements must not be considered separately, but rather as equal parts of the whole person, with the health of all three essential to well-being.

Health must be integrated into education as a primary component of a child's preparation for life. Eating habits, food selections, exercising programs, addictive substances, and harmful life-style practices must be explained in detail so that an informed student body can move on to become an action-oriented adult population capable of making good health decisions. Role models are important. Teachers, as well as health providers, must look to their own eating, exercise, and emotional health patterns so that students witness the relationship between the rhetoric and vision of health, and the day-to-day practices that make good health a reality.

Health and health care should be elevated as a public priority to a way of life. Education, which is fundamental to our nation's ability to thrive as a world leader, can incorporate the health component in such a way that it is not a separate, auxiliary, or elective course.

DRIVEN BY PRIVATE SECTOR

History has shown that in the U.S., the federal government is most effective in directing defense and public safety efforts and protecting the rights of society. It is less effective in delivering services or in paying for services that are rendered on an individual basis. Inevitably, the personal side of these services takes a back seat to the economic pressures and priorities of government. The writers of the Constitution envisioned a role of government that was supportive of society, not operative in society.

Government is generally inefficient when personal interaction is the foundation for the delivery of services. Based on the experience of other nations, it is clear that those health systems created and run by governments become stagnant over time. Individual incentives and the drive for innovation are often lost in the red tape and minutia that result from bureaucratic micromanagement. Goals and the big picture get lost in attempts to control expenditures and behavior through the regulatory process.

The private sector is making changes in many parts of the country. Evolutionary reform is well underway, led by states such as California and Minnesota. For more than two decades, the health system has been changing at an increasing rate. The phrase "managed care" is used to describe many of the delivery options which have emerged. In summary, three generations of managed care can be identified. While each generation has unique characteristics, some of which have not been achieved, they illustrate the profound changes.

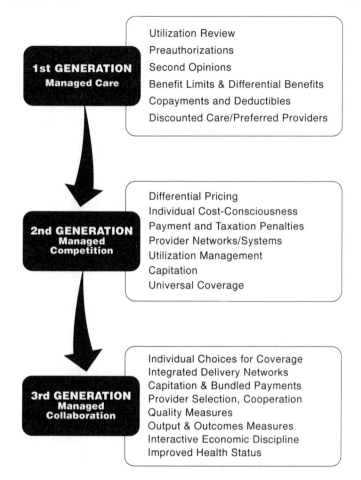

1st GENERATION
Managed Care

Utilization Review
Preauthorizations
Second Opinions
Benefit Limits & Differential Benefits
Copayments and Deductibles
Discounted Care/Preferred Providers

2nd GENERATION
Managed
Competition

Differential Pricing
Individual Cost-Consciousness
Payment and Taxation Penalties
Provider Networks/Systems
Utilization Management
Capitation
Universal Coverage

3rd GENERATION
Managed
Collaboration

Individual Choices for Coverage
Integrated Delivery Networks
Capitation & Bundled Payments
Provider Selection, Cooperation
Quality Measures
Output & Outcomes Measures
Interactive Economic Discipline
Improved Health Status

A PEOPLE-BASED SYSTEM

Health care's new order for the twenty-first century must be a people-based system that relies on the ingenuity and motivations of private citizens who share a common mission. The previous chapters discussed the importance of bundled and capitated payments to providers in an integrated network. Through aggregated payments and the elimination of the do-more-to-make-more mentality, emphasis can be placed on improving health status so that everybody will benefit.

The system should be designed to foster and support innovation and productivity, freeing the system of obstacles we have come to accept. Primary among these is the current legal morass, which serves only to thwart these new developments by feeding off of old practices and standards that are inconsistent with the newly emerging values.

TORT REFORM

Costly defensive medicine and other actions taken to protect providers against a litigious society must be eliminated. With 43 percent more lawyers than physicians, it is highly likely that defensive medicine will continue until a framework is established that eliminates the potential for obstreperous litigation.

A national floor for state tort reforms is needed. Based on the experiences of several states during the past twenty years, we know that certain reforms produce demonstrable savings while protecting the public interest.

Several states have enacted tort reforms, but California produced the best proven combination of laws. In 1975, malpractice premiums for California hospitals and physicians were the highest in the nation. A crisis existed.

The California Legislature enacted several laws in 1975, called the Medical Injury Compensation Reform Act (MICRA). The major provisions of MICRA and a 1988 referendum are:

1) A cap on noneconomic loss, (i.e., pain and suffering)
2) A sliding scale limitation on plaintiff lawyers' contingency fees

3) Disclosure of collateral recovery sources (to discourage double recoveries)
4) Periodic payment of large settlements or judgements
5) Proportionate assignment of liability for non-economic losses on the basis of degree of fault
6) Reasonable statute of limitations

Hospital and physician malpractice premiums in California today are well below the 1975 peak. Yet, by all measurement methodologies so far devised, the quality of health care in California has not suffered. These, or similar provisions, can be applied on a federal level and should form the core of nationwide reform.

Clearly, actual economic losses, such as past and future earnings and health care costs, should be fully recoverable. Further, effective licensing and discipline laws pertaining to health care providers are essential. But, the runaway lottery-driven lawsuits and their impact on rising health care costs must be dealt with in the context of health care reform. Federally directed, tort reform standards administered by the states are a workable starting point.

ERISA

Another obstacle to building the new order is the federal Employment Retirement Income Security Act (ERISA). It was enacted in 1976 to establish standards for employers that provide self-insured benefits, such as pensions and health care for employees and to guarantee solvency of plans—an effort that should continue to be promoted.

However, ERISA preempts states from regulating employer-directed plans that are covered by the law. Since health care coverage is an ERISA "benefit," states are precluded from including ERISA health plans in their reforms. Thus, a federal change is needed to create consistency nationwide and allow states the latitude to establish uniform health reforms among all employers and employees.

The ERISA law should be modified to fit in with a nationally created system of incentives and responsibilities, creating fiscal stability as well as uniformity and portability for employees to receive health services, irrespective of their place of employment.

PERSONAL CHOICES

If reform is to occur, it is necessary for coordination to take place throughout society; it cannot occur only in the delivery of health services. The new order requires a comprehensive effort, based on the acceptance of a common vision through education, the establishment of a predictable and sound payment and finance base, the reconfiguring of the delivery system to eliminate costly duplication, and ultimately, a greater partnership between providers and users to increase individual accountability for a healthy life-style.

This accountability manifests itself in personal choices within the new model. The checks-and-balance system ensures that individuals have recourse, in the event they are dissatisfied with the price or quality of services. Through the selection of physicians within a network, through outcome reporting and through the ability to change delivery networks on an annual basis, individual choice is assured. With consumer choice driving the system, the parameters and incentives for providers to promote quality, cooperation, communication, economic efficiency, and to place the customer first, are established.

THE COURAGE TO CHANGE

Change in something as vital as health care sets enormous forces in motion. If the dynamics of the change are not understood by everybody, they can seem threatening and disruptive. Like all major life changes, health care reform carries with it a potentially explosive mix of uncertainty and doubt. However, it also contains the solid promise of improving health status and providing high-quality health care to every American at an affordable price.

FILLING THE GAPS AND MEETING SPECIAL CIRCUMSTANCES

The true test of civilization is how it treats its poor and disadvantaged.
—SAMUEL JOHNSON.

It is imperative that seamless health care is provided nationwide. To reach that goal, a safety net must be preserved for those individuals who fall through the cracks or choose to participate in the system only when they require immediate care. These disenfranchised and underserved populations are often homeless, underemployed, undocumented immigrants, or persons who may not have the mental capacity to join the system on their own. Society, nevertheless, has a responsibility to provide for those who cannot provide for themselves. Society also has a duty to educate and create incentives for those who consciously choose not be a part of the program.

FINANCIAL CHALLENGE

Those not enrolled in a health plan present a financial challenge to the delivery network because no income is generated for the services they require. This problem is compounded by the fact that they also will not benefit from the many services designed to promote healthy life-styles and behaviors. As a result, this population often requires expensive services at the point of entry, which is often the hospital emergency room.

A major portion of this population are the undocu-mented immigrants. Growing by several hundred thou-sand people annually, this population presents specific problems for states such as California, Texas, New York, Illinois, Florida, and New Jersey, which receive a dispro-portionate share of immigrants. More than 50 percent of all immigrants that illegally enter the U.S end up in Cali-fornia.

The first step toward alleviating the problem is to lift the burden of health treatment from these states. Undocu-mented immigrants enter the U.S. in violation of federal laws, and are able to do so because the federal government enforces the laws inadequately. Therefore, this should be seen as a national problem and these individuals should not be the sole responsibility of a single state's employers, providers, or government.

Estimated undocumented immigrants*

United States: Select Years 1980-1993†

Year	Undocumented Immigrants
1980	3,000,000
1990	3,300,000
1991	3,500,000
1992	3,700,000
1993	4,000,000

* Derived from the estimation of the number of undocumented immigrants in the 1980 Census, various national surveys and administrative data on undocumented immigrants who applied for amnesty under the Immigration Reform and Control Act (IRCA) of 1986.

† The IRCA proclaimed amnesty to immigrants who were in the United States. The results of this act are shown in the substantial number of immigrants between 1990 and 1993.

SOURCE: Unofficial estimates, Population Analysis and Evaluation Staff, Population Division, Bureau of the Census, Washington, D.C., 1993.

Disproportionate undocumented immigrant* population states

1993

Rank	State	Total Undocumented Immigrant Population	Percent of Total U.S. Immigrant Population
1	California	2,083,000	52.1%
2	Texas	521,000	13.0
3	New York	371,000	9.3
4	Illinois	270,000	6.7
5	Florida	137,000	3.4
6	New Jersey	70,000	1.7

* Derived from the estimates of undocumented immigrants in the 1980 Census; various national surveys and administrative data on undocumented aliens who applied for amnesty under the Immigration Reform and Control Act (IRCA) of 1986.

SOURCE: Unofficial estimates, Population Analysis and Evaluation Staff, Population Division, Bureau of the Census, Washington D.C., 1993.

At the same time, it must be recognized that many undocumented immigrants come to the U.S. unemployed and seeking health care. While the U.S. may have a heart as big as the world, our pocketbook is so inadequate that now we are failing to pay for the needs of legal residents.

That economic reality must be recognized. As a part of its responsibilities to protect our society, government must effectively enforce the immigration laws.

Under any circumstances, there will continue to be patients who fall through the cracks and require services. As politically unpopular as it might be, it is essential that the federal government allocate the financial resources to pay providers who render services to those outside the system.

FUNDING THE SAFETY NET

One proposed funding method is a surcharge on employers and employees. However, to place this burden specifically on employers and employees is inconsistent with the objective to spread the financial responsibility throughout society—especially when the obligation clearly rests with the entire nation. More appropriately, this responsibility should be funded by general revenues. Employers will be shouldering the burden of at least 80 percent of those who now are uninsured.

We must avoid the temptation to assume that savings will start accruing at the point of initial implementation. It will take several years for patients, providers and others to adjust fully to the changes. If funds to the safety net and disproportionate share hospitals are cut back, these vulnerable institutions will not survive.

PART-TIME AND SEASONAL EMPLOYEES

Employer-based coverage for part-time employees should be based on a formula whereby employers pay a proportion of the per-worker premium based on the ratio of hours worked to a thirty hour work week.

RURAL AREAS

Populations living outside urban spheres of influence present special circumstances. The lack of a critical mass of people living in these areas often makes it impossible for a comprehensive set of benefits to be delivered locally. Most rural communities are able to provide the primary and secondary services that people require, usually at least 80 percent of the services needed. Moreover, most rural communities have the potential to develop wellness and preventative-practice programs and to generally improve health status.

The payment arrangements in rural areas should be based on the services provided locally. Flexibility is necessary so that capitation, block payments, fee-for-service, and other arrangements can be negotiated. Rural areas, outside of metropolitan statistical areas (MSAs), or rural locations within MSAs, should be designated as swing territories. The rural communities should decide how they wish to organize, which will be either locally on whatever payment basis is negotiated, or in conjunction with a community health network based in an urbanized area. A small proportion of total health care costs are consumed in rural areas. Since it is less expensive to care for people in rural areas than to transport them for primary and most secondary care, special options should be provided. Generally speaking, rural communities and their residents have a greater sense of common purpose and collective well-being than residents in large cities. Thus, it makes sense to extend latitude to rural areas as long as the vision of universal access is not compromised.

Funding for specialized services not available locally can come from two sources. Alliances or carriers for rural patients can either pay on a fee-for-service basis or funding can be generated through the premiums paid to community health networks in rural areas. In either event, allowing remote rural communities to provide as many services and health promotion programs as possible will be less expensive and will produce a higher quality of service than attempting to squeeze them into the urban networks.

HIGH RISK AREAS

The circumstances existing in some inner cities and other underserved areas, also requires special consideration. It is necessary that payments made to delivery systems serving these areas be risk-adjusted and, therefore, recognize the health status of such population groups.

Initially, community health networks that assume the responsibility for people with poorer health status and higher risks should be paid an additional capitation amount to cover the extra needs of the enrollees. Risk-adjusted payments may become unnecessary over time as health status rises to meet that of the general population. Incentives to community health networks that improve health status will encourage this process.

SPECIALTY FACILITIES

Specialized technical and tertiary services are not used as much as primary and secondary services, and, therefore, may not be a necessary component of every network. It may not be logistically or financially feasible, for example, for each network to offer children's or teaching hospitals, trauma centers, burn units, transplantation programs, certain rehabilitative facilities, or other unique services.

However, it is necessary that all of these services be available to enrollees of each network. Specialized services could be made available on a contract basis or through capitation payments. The networks and delivery systems could receive, through their capitation payments, monies for these services. Each network, in turn, would then contract with the specialty institutions. It becomes, thus, a cooperative venture among competing networks, just as competing stores in a shopping center contribute to pay for common-area maintenance, parking, insurance, etc. In this way, a community interest in the quality of specialty care is established, setting forth strong incentives for the specialty providers to be efficient and cooperative. Providing specialty services in a cost-effective manner that minimizes the duplication of expensive technology works to the advantage of all parties.

Some networks may be located in densely populated areas where a sufficient population base requires the specialty services in a volume that becomes cost effective. In these cases, it will be in the best interests of the networks to provide those services themselves. Funds for teaching health professions to provide these services still would be required in such instances.

It is possible that states may choose to meet this challenge in different ways, possibly by blending the outlined approaches. The important point is that within the bottom-up, capitation-generated budgets, funding must be provided to meet the special circumstances presented by rural areas, safety net providers, and specialty institutions.

FLEXIBLE PROGRAMS

Filling the gaps can be viewed as a monumental problem
or it can be managed as a regular way of doing business.
Building a new order for the delivery of health care
requires that a system be established that addresses the
vast majority of circumstances and needs. It further
requires that a supplemental program be established to
deal with those populations that do not fit the mainstream mold.

We can meet the special circumstances and fill the
gaps in health care with decisive action from our policy
makers. Whatever the specifics, these actions must be
compatible with the underlying incentives of the new
paradigm, and they must be based on a realistic evaluation
of what we can and cannot expect from our health care
system.

PUTTING IT TOGETHER

Managed collaboration is the term used to describe the
plan which is suggested. It may seem like an oxymoron
at first blush, but a closer look reveals a concept of order
built upon a foundation of team responses to incentives
which produce positive behavioral changes.

A key to the success of managed collaboration is real
integration. This means that the community health plan
and providers should be consolidated into an organiza-
tional entity which shares a common vision, goals and
financial incentives. Major providers must have congruent, interdependent incentives to achieve long-term economic discipline. The most practical payment methods to
accomplish this are capitation or bundled payments. Economic discipline is achieved through the aggregation of

the negotiations between alliances, employers and the community health plans. Since all premiums to the alliances and all payments to community health plans are capitated or bundled, a fixed, annual expenditure level will be determined. This bottom-up approach is more responsive to local needs and circumstances than a formula-driven top-down premium or payment cap.

The following exhibits show the transitional and mature phases of managed collaboration.

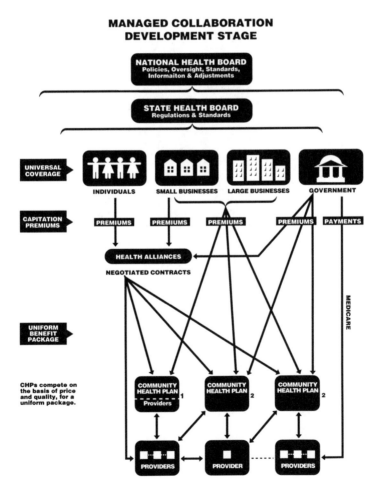

MANAGED COLLABORATION DEVELOPMENT STAGE

MANAGED COLLABORATION
MATURE STAGE

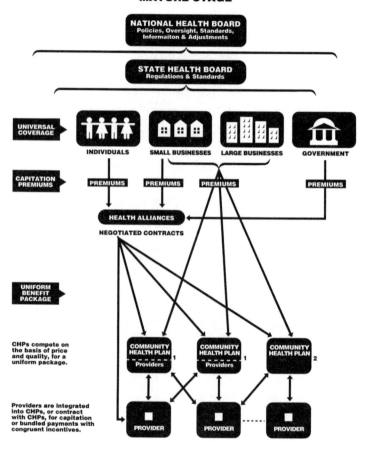

1 – integrated CHP
2 – insurance carrier CHP

BLAZING THE TRAIL

▼

Transforming the new paradigm from concept to working reality requires two crucial elements. First, the process must be championed by leaders with the ability to develop and share a clearly defined sense of direction and mission—a vision of the desired future. Second, the American public must take ownership of that vision. People must believe in the goals and strategies of the new model so intensely that they are willing to take measures to see that the vision becomes a reality. Without the majority's intellectual and emotional "buy-in," health care reform will have little chance for success.

Leadership must be consistent and free from divisive political partisanship. Putting priorities into place requires more than political rhetoric; it requires a bipartisan effort that inspires acceptance and incites public participation.

SIDESTEPPING PITFALLS

Two major mistakes must be avoided throughout the process. The first is the impulse by federal government to commandeer the plan's implementation. The hearts and minds of the American public would be lost in a federally orchestrated prescribed command-and-control approach. Although a majority of Americans believe that significant health care reform is needed, there is widespread skepticism that the federal government can solve the problem. While the federal government should play the major role in establishing the policies for universal access, the uniform benefit package, provider and patient incentives, economic discipline, and implementation of the new model should be carried out at the local level, in partnership with the private sector. As the states exert compatible leadership, it is likely that public opinion will coalesce and support the tough decisions that must be made to realize the vision.

The second pitfall we must avoid is assuming that the new paradigm can be achieved overnight. The existing structure is the result of 200 years of development and it is unrealistic to assume it can be changed in a short time. What lies ahead is one of the most substantial and important social changes of the past 100 years. The social, political, financial, moral, and ethical changes that are necessary require more than a casual passing of a law. Government, employers, employees, providers, and the general public must understand, accept, and buy into the philosophy and vision of the new paradigm. It will take at least a decade to put the proper policies and structures into place, and even longer to achieve the sociological changes.

THE ESSENTIAL PUBLIC DEBATE

It is essential that the transition to the new delivery, financing, and payment system involve public debate. People must know that they have played an active part in its definition and implementation. They must also believe that any sacrifices must be made for the common good and that no individuals are being arbitrarily disadvantaged.

The idea that additional money is initially required for the system must be accepted in the context of our social responsibilities and weighed against the consequences of inaction. Because it is the highest in the world, the escalating cost of health care is already hampering American businesses in global competition.

Rising health care costs have an inflationary value as employers are forced to raise product and service prices to cover employee health coverage plans. Individuals who are artificially protected from health care costs through third-party carriers may be concerned about the direct costs of the new system, but the alternative—allowing health care costs to be shifted at exponential rates—must be recognized as a pathway to economic disaster.

LEADERSHIP DURING CHANGE

Although health care reform is deemed necessary by a
public majority, the mandate for reform is tempered by
uncertainty over how that reform may jeopardize existing
coverage. Moreover, when change does occur, there will be
a certain amount of uncertainty as old ways are aban-
doned and new ones implemented. To be successful, leaders must recognize these conditions and allay public fears,
both before and during the transition.

All major change produces anxiety as known quanti-
ties give way to unknown ones. To reduce the apprehen-
sion that many will feel during this transition, the status
quo regarding quality and access should be preserved as
much as possible. This means that short-term, arbitrary
regulations, such as price controls and other restrictions,
should be avoided. While temporary problems will arise
during this transition period, government leaders must
allow time for innovative approaches to solve them.

CHANGE REQUIRES COMMITMENT

It is essential that all parties understand that the overhaul
of the health care system will require a commitment of
time, money, and energy. It will require the creation of a
different type of infrastructure, which will not evolve easily or painlessly. The entire process will demand a strong
sense of commitment, based on a thorough understanding
of the stated goals, from all those involved.

With that in mind, it is essential that a nationwide
public debate be encouraged. All of the concepts in this
book—from the capitated payment and financing process,
to the system of collaborative competition, as well as other
proposed solutions—must be laid before the public and

discussed. To the extent possible, they must be discussed with one issue in mind: will they, taken as a whole over the long term, produce accessible, affordable, quality health care for all Americans?

A UNIFIED EFFORT

Inherent in the formation of policy must be the blending of personal interests and social responsibility. At the same time, polls continuously illustrate that the public believes that the private system—driven by competition, innovation, and initiative—is superior to one controlled by government. This underlying belief in a market-based system lays the groundwork for pursuing a managed-collaboration philosophy, which serves both private and social goals.

LONG-TERM APPROACH

Because the transition process will most likely take several years, it is important that the plan be promoted as a long-term solution. Incremental goals and milestones should be developed to monitor progress. As each goal is met, the progress should be reported to the public. This will help underscore public trust during the uncertainty of the transition period. It will also encourage continued discipline among the stakeholders in the new financing, payment, and delivery systems.

Visibly marking the progress of the plan is crucial. In a society where problems are "solved" in eight-second sound bites, the trend is toward quick fixes and fast assignments of blame. We know these do not work. To minimize the uncertainty, stakeholders must be constantly apprised of the plan's progress during transition. It is essential that a specific proposal be advocated and that the blueprint lay out the benchmarks and goals to be accomplished.

FOCUS ON QUALITY

An essential ingredient to successful long-term reform is the ability of the provider community to incorporate total-quality-management (TQM) and continuous-quality-improvement (CQI) principles and actions into their lives and everyday conduct. Quality is the competitive advantage that brings reality to the vision.

The change to TQM requires a commitment from providers to build long-term relationships with patients. Successful providers in the new paradigm must commit themselves 100 percent to service, customer satisfaction, and quality improvement.

The most powerful framework for pursuing success under the new paradigm is through a complete commitment to total quality improvement. This requires a new vision by providers. Indeed, a growing number of hospitals and health care systems are already implementing CQI measures to combat escalating costs, decreased occupancy rates, dwindling reimbursements, and intense competition for qualified staff. The future, however, demands that all providers define, or redefine their personal missions to include a commitment to complete customer satisfaction, 100 percent of the time. While this may not be an obtainable goal, it is an enormously powerful vision.

The adage that, "The main thing is keeping the main thing the main thing," hits the nail squarely on the head. With our eyes on the vision, our intellect on the plan, and our hearts given over to the quest for quality, we can keep the main thing the main thing—and health care reform will be realized.

SEIZE THE DAY

The time has never been better to make a change. The current state of crisis within health care has one broad silver lining. It has focused public attention on the big picture: the need to rebuild the system toward granting full accessibility at an affordable rate. For decisionmakers, this translates into a unique window of opportunity to make serious and substantial changes. The public has already expressed its readiness to back such a plan—as long as it is based on common sense, does not include governmental takeover, and does not jeopardize their current coverage.

The environment that exists today may not present itself again for decades. To squander this unique opportunity for health reform could be considered one of the great failures of the twentieth century.

THE HEALTH REFORM SEASON

On September 22, 1993, President Bill Clinton unveiled the tenants of the Administration's health reform plan. The six principles of the plan are: security, simplicity, savings, choice, quality, and responsibility. This foundation is supported by a comprehensive proposal that falls within the general category of managed competition. Many of the concepts in the president's plan and the managed collaboration model are similar. Some differences exist, the most significant of which are: top-down formula-driven budget controls versus bottom-up economic discipline, majority enrollment in health alliances versus balanced alliance-employer coverage, and choice versus emphasis on capitated payments to integrated community health networks.

The president has demonstrated an unprecedented commitment to health reform. Many members of the Congress also have sponsored reform bills. Several providers groups and others have proposed reform plans. All of these models have merit and deserve full debate. It is encouraging to see leadership from all sides of the political spectrum and a growing willingness to work out a compromise which can be enacted into law.

Regardless of the plan which ultimately is passed, moving to universal access and bringing economic discipline to health care will be a monumental accomplishment. Philosophies and preferences aside, we must not let this opportunity pass.

AFTERWORD

▼

The public imperative for health care reform is undeniable. Making it happen, however, will require leadership at all levels. Elected officials and leaders from organizations representing providers, business, labor, and consumers, must work together toward the common goal. While federal officials must look toward state governments to support the process, the states in turn, must look to private leadership.

Assuming a federal reform proposal and implementation strategy is enacted, coalitions of interested parties at the state level must be formed to carry out regional plans that are consistent with the national plan and address special statewide issues. The challenge is to allow states the opportunity to prepare a plan that is tailored to the local flavor of their communities, within the national policy.

It is unlikely that a federal system, based on a top-down approach to control expenditures, can meet the same standards of health care as a decentralized, locally controlled effort. However, nationwide standards are necessary for all players if the regional and local models are to maintain the integrity of the national program.

Throughout the process, it is essential that we keep in mind that managed collaboration is not the destination of health care reform. Rather, it is the vehicle used to achieve the real vision of universal access to a uniform benefit package, delivered with appropriate quality and driven by economic discipline.

Quality knows no fear and the human intellect is limitless. Both of these axioms will be tested during the health reform debate. The conceptual logic of a collaboration model, combined with the practical way ideals and human motivations are integrated, will overcome obstacles that otherwise could cause them to collapse.

In the end, the new paradigm should be driven by a clear vision based on the concept that equitable access to quality health care is every person's right. That vision is obtainable, if we are willing to act now and do the right thing. For those who have the courage to trust in the vision, the reward is clear: a legacy of health that will last far into the next century.

BIBLIOGRAPHY

Abel-Smith, B., "Cost Containment and New Priorities in the European Community," The Milbank Quarterly, Vol. 70, No. 3, 1992: 393–422.

American Heart Association, Heart and Stroke Facts, 1988–1993, Dallas, 1988–1993.

American Hospital Association, Annual Hospital Survey, 1972–1992, Chicago, 1973–1992.

American Hospital Association, Hospital Statistics, 1975–1992, Chicago, 1976–1992.

American Hospital Association, Hospitals Guide Issue, 1957–1970, Chicago, 1958–1970.

American Hospital Association, Selected Hospital Statistics, 1982–1991; Statistical Profile, Chicago, 1992.

American Medical Association, Socioeconomic Characteristics of Medical Practice, Chicago, 1993.

Amler, R., and H. B. Dull, "Closing the Gap: The Burden of Unnecessary Illness," Oxford University Press, N.Y., 1987.

Anderson, G. F., R. Heyssel, and R. Dickler, "Competition vs. Regulation: Its Effect on Hospitals," Health Affairs, Vol. 12, No. 1, 1993: 70–80.

Barker, D. K., "The Effects of Tort Reform on Medical Malpractice Insurance Markets: An Empirical Analysis," Journal of Health Politics, Policy, and Law, Vol. 17, No. 1, 1992: 143–161.

Beauchamp, D. E., "Waiting for the Big One: Confessions of a Policy Surfer Looking for the Universal Health Care Wave," Journal of Health Politics, Policy, and Law, Vol. 18, No. 1, 1993: 203–228.

Berken, A., M.D., "America's Med-Life Crisis: Urgent Problems, Revolutionary Solutions," QUON Publishing, Garden City, N.Y., 1993.

Buck, J. A., and M. S. Kamlet, "Problems with Expanding Medicaid for the Uninsured," Journal of Health Politics, Policy, and Law, Vol. 18, No. 1, 1993: 1–25.

Burner, S. T., et al., "National Health Expenditures Through 2030," Health Care Financing Review, Vol. 14, No. 1, 1992.

California Medical Association, Physicians and Health Care Statistics, San Francisco, 1981.

Congress of the United States, "Economic Implications of Rising Health Care Costs," Congressional Budget Office, Oct. 1992.

Culyer, A. J., and A. Meads, "The United Kingdom: Effective, Efficient, Equitable?," Journal of Health Politics, Policy, and Law, Vol. 17, No. 4, 1992: 667–688.

Durenberger, D., "Perspective: Government and the Competitive Marketplace," Health Affairs, Vol. 12, No. 1, 1993: 81–84.

Edwards, J. N., R. J. Blendon, R. Leitman, E. Morrison, I. Morrison, and H. Taylor, "DataWatch: Small Business and the National Health Care Reform Debate," Health Affairs, Vol. 11, No. 1, 1992: 164–173.

Employee Benefit Research Institute, "Sources of Health Insurance and Characteristics of the Uninsured," EBRI Special Report, Issue Brief No. 133, Washington, D.C., Jan. 1993.

Enthoven, A. C., "The History and Principles of Managed Competition," Health Affairs, Vol. 12, Supplement, 1993: 24–48.

Enthoven, A. C., "Managed Competition: An Agenda for Action," Health Affairs, Vol. 7, No. 3, 1988: 25–47.

Etheredge, L., and S. Jones, "Commentary: Managing a Pluralist Health System," Health Affairs, Vol. 10, No. 4, 1991: 93–105.

Evans, R. G., "Canada: The Real Issues," Journal of Health Politics, Policy, and Law, Vol. 17, No. 4, 1992: 739–762.

Fuchs, V. R., "National Health Insurance Revisited," Health Affairs, Vol. 10, No. 4, 1991: 7–17.

Fuchs, V. R., "The 'Competition Revolution' in Health Care," Health Affairs, Vol. 7, No. 3, 1988: 5–24.

Gauthier, A. K., D. L. Rogal, N. L. Barrand, and A. B. Cohen, "Administrative Costs in the U.S. Health Care System: The Problem or the Solution?," Inquiry: The Journal of Health Care

Organization, Provision, and Financing, Vol. 29, No. 3, 1992: 308–320.

Grogan, C. M., "Deciding on Access and Levels of Care: A Comparison of Canada, Britain, Germany, and the United States," Journal of Health Politics, Policy, and Law, Vol. 17, No. 2, 1992: 213–232.

Health Insurance Association of America, Source Book of Health Insurance Data, 1991, Washington, D.C., 1992.

Hillman, A. L., W. R. Greer, and N. Goldfarb, "Safeguarding Quality in Managed Competition," Health Affairs, Vol. 12, Supplement, 1993: 110–122.

Ikegami, N., "Japan: Maintaining Equity through Regulated Fees," Journal of Health Politics, Policy, and Law, Vol. 17, No. 4, 1992: 689–714.

Kronick, R., "Where Should the Buck Stop: Federal and State Responsibilities in Health Care Financing Reform," Health Affairs, Vol. 12, Supplement, 1993: 87–98.

Letsch, S. W., et al., "National Health Expenditures, 1991," Health Care Financing Review, Vol. 14, No. 2, 1992.

Mendelson, D. N., and W. B. Schwartz, "The Effects of Aging and Population Growth on Health Care Costs," Health Affairs, Vol. 12, No. 1, 1993: 119–125.

Miller, R. H., and H. S. Luft, "Perspective: Diversity and Transition in Insurance," Health Affairs, Vol. 10, No. 4, 1991: 37–47.

Moran, D. W., and P. R. Wolfe, "Can Managed Care Control Costs?," Health Affairs, Vol. 10, No. 4, 1991: 120–128.

National Center for Health Statistics, "Advance Report of Final Mortality," Monthly Vital Statistics Report, Vol. 41, No. 7, 1993.

National Center for Health Statistics, "Annual Summary, Birth, Deaths, Marriages: US, 1980, 1985 and 1990," Monthly Vital Statistics Report, Vol. 40, No. 13, 1981–1993.

National Center for Health Statistics, Vital Statistics of the United States, 1973, Volume II Mortality, Parts A & B, 1975.

National Center for Health Statistics, Vital Statistics of the United States, 1975, Volume II Mortality, Parts A & B, 1977.

Newhouse, J. P., "An Iconoclastic View of Health Cost Containment," Health Affairs, Vol. 12, Supplement, 1993: 152–171.

Organization for Economic Cooperation and Development, OECD Health Systems: Facts and Trends, Paris, 1993.

Pauly, M., P. Danzon, P. Feldstein, and J. Hoff, "A Plan for 'Responsible National Health Insurance'," Health Affairs, Vol. 10, No. 1, 1991: 5–25.

Priester, R., "A Values Framework for Health System Reform," Health Affairs, Vol. 11, No. 1, 1992: 84–107.

Reinhardt, U. E., "The United States: Breakthroughs and Waste," Journal of Health Politics, Policy, and Law, Vol. 17, No. 4, 1992: 637–666.

Robinson, J. C., "A Payment Method for Health Insurance Purchasing Cooperatives," Health Affairs, Vol. 12, Supplement, 1993: 65–75.

Schieber, G. J., et al, "Data Watch: Health Spending, Delivery and Outcomes in OECD Countries," Health Affairs, Vol. 12, No. 2, 1993.

Schieber, G. J., et al, "International Health Care Expenditure Trends: 1987," Health Affairs, Vol. 8, No. 3, 1989.

Schulenberg, J.-M.G.v.d., "Germany: Solidarity at a Price," Journal of Health Politics, Policy, and Law, Vol. 17, No. 4, 1992: 715–738.

Sheils, J. F., G. J. Young, and R. J. Rubin, "O Canada: Do We Expect Too Much from Its Health System?," Health Affairs, Vol. 11, No. 1, 1992: 7–20.

Shortell, S. M., "A Model for State Health Care Reform," Health Affairs, Vol. 11, No. 1, 1992: 108–127.

Sparer, M. S., "States in a Reformed Health System: Lessons from Nursing Home Policy," Health Affairs, Vol. 12, No. 1, 1993: 7–20.

Spencer, G., "Projections of the Population of the United States by Age, Sex, and Race: 1988 to 2080," Bureau of the Census, U.S. Department of Commerce, P. 25, No. 1018, 1988.

St. Paul Marine and Fire Insurance Company, "Hospitals Update," The St. Paul's 1991–1993 Annual Report to Policyholders, St. Paul, 1993.

Starr, P., "Design of Health Insurance Purchasing Cooperatives," Health Affairs, Vol. 12, Supplement, 1993: 58–64.

Starr, P., and W. A. Zelman, "A Bridge to Compromise: Competition under a Budget," Health Affairs, Vol. 12, Supplement, 1993: 7–23.

Tallon, J. R., Jr., and R. P. Nathan, "Federal/State Partnership for Health System Reform," Health Affairs, Vol. 11, No. 4, 1992: 7–16.

United States Bureau of the Census, Historical Statistics of the United States, Colonial Times to 1957, Washington, D.C., 1960.

United States Bureau of the Census, Population Analysis and Evaluation Staff, Population Division, Washington, D.C., 1993, Unofficial Estimates.

United States General Accounting Office, "Access to Health Care: States Respond to Growing Crisis," GAO/HRD-92-70, June 1992.

United States General Accounting Office, "Canadian Health Insurance: Lessons for the United States," GAO/HRD-91-90, June 1991.

United States General Accounting Office, "Health Care Spending: Nonpolicy Factors Account for Most State Differences," GAO/HRD-92-36, Feb. 1992.

United States General Accounting Office, "Health Care Spending Control: The Experience of France, Germany, and Japan," GAO/HRD-92-9, Nov. 1991.

United States General Accounting Office, "U.S. Health Care Spending: Trends, Contributing Factors, and Proposals for Reform," GAO/HRD-91-102, June 1991.

Weiner, J. P., and G. de Lissovoy, "Razing a Tower of Babel: A Taxonomy for Managed Care and Health Insurance Plans," Journal of Health Politics, Policy, and Law, Vol. 18, No. 1, 1993: 75–104.

Zelman, W. A., "Who Should Govern the Purchasing Cooperative?," Health Affairs, Vol. 12, Supplement, 1993: 49–57.

INDEX